A

SUSAN HOLMES

Second Edition

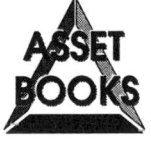

ASSET BOOKS LTD., DORKING, SURREY RH4 2TU, UNITED KINGDOM

Asset Books Ltd
1 Paper Mews, 330 High Street,
Dorking, Surrey RH4 2TU

First published in 1988 by Austen Cornish Ltd in association with
the Lisa Sainsbury Foundation

This edition published in 1996 by Asset Books Ltd

A catalogue record for this book is available from the British Library.

ISBN 1 9001 79 10 5

Printed and bound in Great Britain by Hobbs the Printer Ltd

CONTENTS

PREFACE

The aim of this book is to provide the fundamental principles underlying the use of radiation as a therapeutic entity in the treatment of malignant disease. Although specific techniques are discussed at times throughout, not all units will follow exactly the same policy with regard to the techniques employed in the radiotherapeutic approach to treatment so that readers are advised to check on local policy with regard to the procedures employed.

Throughout this book the female gender has been used to refer to nurses, and other health care practitioners, of both sexes and the male gender to describe the patient, unless specific examples require otherwise.

Neither the Publishers nor the Author wish to offend or in any other way discriminate against either male health care professionals or female patients but have chosen to use this convention so as to avoid the cumbersome use of gender whenever a nurse or patient is discussed. This system has been chosen since, at present, the majority of health care workers in the UK, particularly nurses, are women.

Susan Holmes
Leatherhead, Surrey
July 1996

INTRODUCTION

Radiotherapy relies on the use of ionising radiation to destroy malignant cell populations. It is one of several possible treatments for cancer yet is used to treat over 50% of all cancer patients at some stage of their disease. It may be the primary form of treatment or be used in conjunction with surgery, chemotherapy or both and be used with either curative or palliative intent.

Radiotherapy may be administered externally (teletherapy) or internally (brachytherapy) the choice being dependent on the type, location and extent of the tumour. It is also influenced by current thinking regarding treatment of the particular tumour type.

Patients facing this type of treatment are often very vulnerable. Many have a fear of radiation which is based, in part at least, on 'old wives' tales' and also on its association with nuclear technology both of which may raise considerable anxiety and concern. In addition, the use OF radiotherapy may confirm the diagnosis of cancer and be viewed as a 'last resort'.

As a method of treatment radiotherapy can neither be seen or felt but it may cause considerable discomfort which can be difficult to understand. It is not, therefore, surprising that many fears and misconceptions exist about the use of radiation as a therapeutic modality. Such feelings are not, unfortunately, restricted only to the patient but are commonly shared by his family and friends and, surprisingly, by members of the health care team despite the wide spread use of radiation in medical practice.

Care cannot be successfully achieved unless the carers themselves understand the principles underlying this method of treatment. This book sets out to provide these principles before moving on to consider its applications in the treatment of malignant disease. The implications for patients are discussed and guideline for care are provided.

CHAPTER 1   HISTORICAL PERSPECTIVE

The use of ionising radiation as a therapeutic modality dates back to the discovery of X-rays by Roentgen in 1895 and radioactivity by Becquerel in the following year; the subsequent isolation of radium by the Curies in 1896 intensified interest still further. It was soon recognised that radiation produced dramatic effects on body tissues and it was not, therefore, surprising that radiation was pronounced a 'cure' for all previously incurable diseases.

When it was realised that radiation could result in marked biological effects, most of which were undesirable, a predictable counter-reaction resulted in claims that radiation had no demonstrable beneficial effects. Subsequent evaluation, after continued and traumatic clinical trials over many years, suggests that radiation differs little from any other medical agent in that it is uniquely beneficial under selected circumstances, such as its use in the treatment of malignant disease.

To reach this point, however, radiation has suffered many uses and abuses and its gestation period as a therapeutic entity has been long and painful. Initially, since surgeons most commonly treated cancer, irradiation was used in single, massive doses to '... produce a slough in lieu of excision' (Bushke, 1970). Not surprisingly this approach had some disastrous consequences as a result of which some, even today, regard radiotherapy with suspicion. Despite this, attempts to harness its use in the treatment of disease have long been reported (Case, 1958) although, in the early stages, the techniques of application were inconsistent and largely non-reproducible. However, reports of its use in the treatment of carcinoma of the stomach (Despeignes, 1896), breast cancer (Grubbe, 1933) and many other physical conditions suggested that radiation could be beneficial when selectively applied. Continued studies of this kind suggested that the use of radiation was most beneficial in the treatment of cancer and the non-reproducibility of the early work suggested that clearly defined conditions and techniques of application were essential.

At this stage, although biological understanding lagged behind technological advances, new techniques were developed and the methods of use explored. In 1913, the first X-ray tube was developed (Coolidge and Charleston, 1950) laying the foundations of external

X-ray therapy. By 1922 this had been further developed and 'deep X-ray therapy' was born (Coolidge and Charleston, 1950). During this period, uterine disease was treated using containers holding radium which were inserted into the uterus; similar techniques were used to treat other interstitial diseases (Cleaves, 1903; Abbé, 1904). Radium was later developed as a teletherapy source (Quick and Richmond, 1955; Case, 1958).

Developments were then rapid and, in 1922, evidence was presented to the International Congress of Otology showing that radiation could be successfully used to treat advanced laryngeal cancer (Regaud et al, 1922). This meant that physicians became interested in its potential as a therapeutic agent and, as developments became more rapid, a rational philosophy for treatment was established. The aim became destruction of tumours with minimum disruption to normal tissues and the 'protracted fractional method' was developed (Coutard, 1934) which, even today, continues to provide the basis of radiation therapy although, for some fast growing tumours, radiation may be delivered more than once a day (hyperfractionation) (Nias, 1990).

However, most of these developments took place in the absence of a method for quantifying the dose of radiation given. Once this was established it became possible for radiation doses to be accurately calculated and administered from newly developed instruments (see Ch 4). The first X-ray generators were in medical use as early as 1932 (Bushke et al, 1950); later developments led to the appearance of cyclotrons, synchro-cyclotrons, betatrons and linear accelerators. At the same time, radium was largely being replaced as a radioactive source by isotopes such as caesium^{137} and cobalt^{60}.

The principle advances in the use of radiation as a therapeutic entity have, however, occurred since the 1940s (Williams and Thwaites, 1993). Nuclear research, and research in high energy physics, enabled the production of new radionuclides (see Ch 2) a number of which (e.g. ^{60}Co) have been used therapeutically as both sealed and unsealed sources. The technology developed for radar during the second world war led to the development of the linear accelerator, now the most important source of radiotherapy (Williams and Thwaites, 1993).

Concurrent developments were taking place in the clinical field alongside increasing understanding of the effects of radiation on biological tissues (the science of radiobiology - see Ch 3). As scientific understanding increased, clinical observations could be explained and a rationale for treatment methods developed. At the same time, the hazards of radiation - and the need for radiation protection - were also recognised with the effect that tighter controls on both the use of radiation and the dose to which the population as a whole, and staff in particular, might be exposed, were introduced (Ch 2). It meant that treatment areas and equipment were developed with safety in mind; it also permitted the development of methods allowing the remote handling of the sealed radioactive sources used in internal therapy (brachytherapy).

Yet, even as late as 1970, Bushke suggested that radiation therapy was still accepted only with reluctance. Despite the fact that radio-therapy is both well accepted and widely practised in Britain, as well as in Europe and the USA, it seems that its early history and apparent 'mysticism', together with its association with nuclear technology, continue to influence the attitudes of both the general public and some of the health care professionals. Nonetheless, for many localised tumours, radiotherapy provides a high probability of cure and is, undoubtedly, the method of choice (Hall, 1985; Williams and Thwaites, 1993).

Developments in computer technology have been one of the most important influences on the practice of radiotherapy in the last twenty years and computers are now found in all radiotherapy departments (Williams and Thwaites, 1993). For example, computerised systems are now used to control or verify the treatment delivered thus increasing the sophistication with which treatment can be monitored and safety can be ensured. Computer-assisted set-up of treatment allows the machine parameters to be precisely and consistently established (Mayles et al, 1993).

Future Trends

The future for radiotherapy as a treatment for cancer remains bright and is likely to be characterised by continued refinement of treatment techniques in attempts to maximise its therapeutic benefits while reducing the damaging effects on normal tissues. Thus there will be continuing investigation of agents designed to protect normal cells (radioprotectors) and to enhance the radiosensitivity of malignant cells (see Ch 3). The use of multimodality therapy will increase.

Alternative methods of treatment, such as hyperfractionation (Ch 4) will continue to be developed and investigation of ways of potentiating the effects of radiation will continue (e.g. hyperthermia). Heat is, in itself, known to be cytotoxic and controlled hyperthermia, when combined with radiotherapy, will enhance tumour cell kill without excessive damage to adjacent normal cells (Hilderley and Dow, 1992). It is likely that this approach will be further developed.

At the same time, investigation of external therapy, reliant on particulate radiations, such as fast neutrons, protons, negative pi-mesons and heavy ions (see p49) will continue and an increased use of prophylactic intra-operative radiotherapy (IOR) will be seen. Here the tumour-bearing organ is surgically exposed and, following excision of the resectable portion, a single high dose of radiation is delivered directly to the tumour bed (Goldson, 1981). By protecting normal tissues, the dose delivered to the tumour bed can be maximised so that, despite high treatment doses, side-effects are minimised (Kinsella and Sindelar, 1985). Further external beam therapy may be given once recovery from surgery is complete, The maximal approach to IOR will be investigated.

A concurrent increase in the use of targeted therapy, reliant on the development of radiolabelled antibodies, is also likely (Bucholz, 1990) (Ch 12). This approach, dependent on the increasing understanding of immunobiology, has led to the isolation of tumour-specific monoclonal and polyclonal antibodies (e.g. Kohler, 1986; Gallucci, 1987) which, when bound to a radioisotope, can deliver radiation directly to the tumour and its metastases. This, in theory at least, avoids prolonged exposure of healthy cells while delivering toxic doses to the tumour. However, although this approach has considerable potential it is, to date, associated with a number of problems amongst which is the high incidence of side-effects associated with the antibodies themselves. These include fever, chills, urticaria and other rashes, nausea and vomiting, headaches and hypotension (Oldham and Smalley, 1983). Work to resolve these problems is in progress.

Conclusion

There is little doubt that the use of radiation to treat cancer has, indeed, come a long way since its discovery by Roentgen (1895) and Becquerel (1896). Used alone or in conjunction with other approaches to treatment, it plays a central role in anticancer therapy. It also plays an important role in palliative care when it may provide relief from a wide variety of distressing symptoms (see Ch 4 and Ch 13). Potential developments in the knowledge and understanding of radiation, combined with increasing knowledge of both its beneficial and harmful effects, will, undoubtedly, lead to continued improvement in therapeutic approaches.

Alongside such developments has been an increased recognition of the role of health care professionals in the provision of effective care for those undergoing radiotherapy. As a method of treatment, radiation cannot be seen or felt yet causes varying degrees of discomfort that the patient may find difficult to understand. Care is, therefore, directed not only at reducing the impact of side-effects but also towards the provision of support to help the patient cope with the stresses associated with this type of treatment. Education about the purpose of treatment, the method of administration, the prevention of complications and the management of unavoidable local or systemic toxicity is essential.

Health care practitioners must, therefore, understand the physical and biological principles of radiotherapy, the onset and character of common side-effects and the measures that can be taken to ameliorate toxicity. Such understanding will enable them to provide effective physical and psychological care for affected patients.

REFERENCES

Abbé R, 1904, Radium and radioactivity, Yale Medical Journal, June, 433.

Bucholz J, 1990, Radiolabeled antibody therapy. In: Hassey K, Hilderley L (Editors), Nursing Perspectives in Radiation Oncology, Delmar Publishers, New York.

Bushke F, 1970, Radiation therapy: the past, the present, the future, American Journal of Roentgenology, **108**, 236-46.

Bushke F, Cantril ST, Parker HM, 1950, Supervoltage Roentgen Therapy, Charles C Thomas, Illinois.

Bushke F, Parker HM, 1972, Radiation Therapy in Cancer Management, Grune and Stratton, New York.

Case FT, 1958, History of radiation therapy. In: Progress in Radiation Therapy, Volume 1, Bushke F (Editor), Grune and Stratton, New York.

Cleaves M A, 1903, Radium Therapy, Medical Record, **64**, 601-604

Coolidge WD, Charleston EE, 1950, Roentgen ray tubes. In: Glasser O, (Editor), Medical Physics: Year Book, Chicago.

Coutard H, 1934, Principles of X-ray therapy of malignant disease, Lancet **2**, 1-8.

Despeignes V, 1896, Observations on a case of carcinoma of the stomach treated with roentgen rays, Lyon Medicine, July **428**; Aug. **503** (French).

Gallucci BB, 1987, The immune system and cancer, Oncology Nursing Forum, **14**(6), 3-11.

Goldson A, 1981, Past, present, and prospects of intraoperative radiotherapy (IOR), Seminars in Oncology, **8**, 59-64.

Grubbe EH, 1933, Priority in the therapeutic use of X-rays, Radiology, **21**, 156-162.

Hall ES, 1985, Radiation and Life, Pergamon Press, Oxford.

Hilderley L, Dow KH, 1991, Radiation oncology. In: Baird SB, McCorkle R, Grant M (Editors), Cancer Nursing: A Comprehensive Textbook, WB Saunders Co., London.

Kinsella TJ, Sindelar WF, 1986, Newer methods of cancer treatment: intraoperative radiotherapy. In: DeVita VT, Hellman S, Rosenberg SA (Editors), Principles and Practice of Oncology (Second edition), JB Lippincott, Philadelphia.

Kohler G, 1986, Derivation and diversification of monoclonal antibodies, Science, **233**, 1281-1286.

Mayles WPM, Heisig S, Mayles HMO, 1993, Treatment verification and *in vivo* dosimetry. In: Williams JR, Thwaites DI (Editors), Radiotherapy Physics in Practice, Oxford Medical Publications, Oxford.

Nias AWH, 1990, An Introduction to Radiobiology, John Wiley and Sons, Chichester.

Oldham R, Smalley R, 1983, Immunotherapy: the old and the new, Journal of Biological Response Modifiers, **2**, 1-37.

Quick D, Richmond JA, 1955, Preliminary experiences with a 50 gram converging beam radium unit, American Journal of Roentgenology, **74**, 635-650.

Regaud C, Coutard H, Hautant A, 1922, Contribution au trâitement des cancers endolarynges par les rayons-x. X. International Congres de Otologie, 19-22.

Williams JR, Thwaites DI, 1993, Introduction. In: Williams JR, Thwaites DI (Editors), Radiotherapy Physics in Practice, Oxford Medical Publications, Oxford.

CHAPTER 2   FUNDAMENTALS OF RADIATION

Radiotherapy relies on the use of high energy ionising radiation to treat disease. It is primarily used in the treatment of cancer but has, occasionally, been used to treat benign disorders such as hyper-thyroidism. Its use in treating malignant disease relies on the ability of ionising radiation to interact with the atoms and molecules of body cells to produce specific biological effects which cause damage to either intracellular components or the cell environment (see Ch 3).

Radiation is both a naturally occurring and an artificially created phenomenon; its effects on substances with which it comes into contact underlie the principles of its use in treating malignant disease. The implications for patient care are dependent on an under-standing of the principles of radiation. Radiation therapy is based on several physical and biological principles; these are described below.

IONISATION

Two main types of ionising radiation are used to treat cancer: electromagnetic radiation (X-rays and gamma (γ) rays) and particulate radiation (for example, protons, electrons, neutrons and alpha (α) particles). They have in common their ability to cause ionisation within the tissues they penetrate. Such radiation may be generated spontaneously by radioactive elements or artificially created.

Radiation is ionising when it is able to disrupt the chemical structure of material through which it passes causing damage to, or disruption of, the molecules contained by living tissues. Although visible light, radio-waves and ultraviolet light (i.e. sunlight) are also forms of radiation they cannot cause damage through ionisation. However, when large amounts are involved, they too can induce biological change (e.g. sun-burn). Before ionisation can be fully understood it is necessary to review atomic structure.

All living matter comprises molecules the basis of which is the atom. Each atom consists of two parts: the nucleus and the shell(s) (orbits). It can be seen from Figure 2.1 that the nucleus contains protons (positively charged) and neutrons (no electrical charge). The shell contains negatively charged electrons which orbit (circle) the nucleus. Each shell can 'hold' only a certain number of electrons; if this number is exceeded, a second or third shell is established more distant from the nucleus.

Figure 2.1 **Structure of a stable atom**

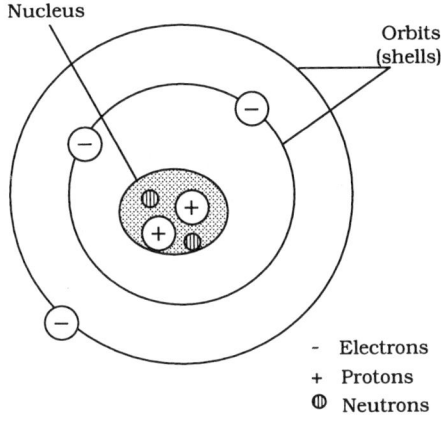

Nucleus

Orbits (shells)

- Electrons
+ Protons
Ⅲ Neutrons

In all atoms, the number of electrons equals the number of protons so that the negative charge is balanced by the positive and the net charge is zero. This is described as a stable atom. In other words, it is the balance between protons and electrons that maintains the stability of an atom.

When an atom carries a charge other than zero it is described as unstable and is said to be an ion. An unstable atom (e.g. radium-226) undergoes breakdown (or decay) (see below) to achieve a more stable state. It is during this process that α, β, or γ rays are emitted.

This process of ionisation should not be confused with the ionised state in which many molecules in aqueous solutions exist under normal chemical conditions (Nias, 1990). This is due to simple dissociation into positively and negatively charged ions which exist in stable equilibrium (for example, water dissociates to produce H^+ and OH^- ions)

Following irradiation, an ion is formed when the energy supplied causes an atom to gain or lose an electron from its orbit around the nucleus; as an electron is ejected from its orbit, energy is released and ionisation occurs. The unstable atom or molecule (group of atoms sharing electrons) and the resultant charged particle (free electron) form highly reactive ion pairs that are capable of further chemical reactions. These physical and chemical changes ultimately lead to cell damage and cell death (see Ch 3). Radiation which is capable of producing ions is described as ionising radiation.

ISOTOPES

Elements are the fundamental substances from which all matter is made (e.g. carbon, hydrogen, oxygen); the nuclei of all atoms of a particular element contain the same number of protons although the number of neutrons may vary. An element is, therefore, made up of many isotopes all of which have the same number of protons, and hence, the same atomic number but a different atomic weight (number of protons and neutrons). An atom of an element that differs only in its atomic weight is called an *isotope*. Those elements with an atomic weight in excess of 209 are naturally radioactive. Examples include radium and uranium.

A radioactive isotope (*radioisotope*) is naturally unstable and undergoes spontaneous nuclear disintegration (*radioactive decay*) which results in the expulsion of α, β or γ rays or charged particles from the radioactive nucleus(*radionuclide*). As seen above, radioactive nuclides may be naturally occurring; the majority, however, are artificially created by bombarding the atomic nuclei of an element with atomic particles, such as neutrons. Cobalt-60 (^{60}Co) is an example of a radioisotope produced in this way; subsequent nuclear disintegration produces α and β rays.

Radioactive decay, and the expulsion of α, β and γ rays from a radioactive nuclide, occurs at a particular rate from each element. This declines in intensity over time and is described in terms of the *half life* ($t_{1/2}$) which describes the time required for a radioisotope to lose 50% of its radioactivity by decay and is constant for any isotope (Table 2.1).

Table 2.1   **Half life of some therapeutic radioisotopes**

Element	$t_{1/2}$	Type of radiation
Caesium (^{137}Cs)	30.0 years	γ and β
Cobalt (^{60}Co)	5.3 years	γ
Radium (^{226}Ra)	16.0 years	γ
Strontium (^{90}Sr)	28.5 years	β
Gold (^{198}Au)	2.7 days	γ
Iodine (^{131}I)	8.05 days	β and γ
Iridium (^{192}Ir)	74.0 days	γ
Phosphorus (^{32}P)	14.3 days	β
Yttrium (^{90}Y)	64.0 hours	γ

Because most radioisotopes are produced from stable elements exposed to bombardment with neutrons (e.g. Cobalt-60, Phosphorus-32, Gold-198) or by nuclear fission (e.g. Caesium-137) they are often referred to as artificial isotopes to allow them to be distinguished from those which are naturally occurring, such as Radium-226 and Radon-222.

IONISING RADIATION

During radioactive decay nuclear disintegration results in the emission of three types of radiation, X-rays, β rays or γ rays. The collision of radiation with orbiting electrons causes ionisation or excitation within the atoms with which it comes into contact.

However, since atoms are in constant motion, and since there may be a considerable distance between the nucleus and its electrons, radiation may pass through the atom without causing ionisation; it may, instead, cause excitation when an electron is moved into an orbit further away from the nucleus.

Ionising radiation is that which disrupts the atoms and molecules of material through which it passes. This is achieved by delivering energy to the tissues being treated causing stable atoms to gain or lose an electron and producing unstable atoms or molecules (*ions*) capable of further chemical reactions. Radiation causing such effects is classified into two groups: electromagnetic radiation and particulate radiation.

Electromagnetic radiation occurs in many forms which differ only in the length of the waves they produce (Figure 2.2). There is an inverse relationship between wavelength and energy (i.e. the shorter the wavelength the greater the energy it carries). It is the short length, high energy waves (X-rays and γ rays) which cause ionisation and which are used extensively in radiation therapy.

Certain fast moving atomic particles, such as α particles, β particles and protons, are also capable of causing ionisation; these can be distinguished from electromagnetic radiation by their ability to carry an electrical charge (either positive or negative).

The damage caused by radiation is dependent upon the depth to which it can penetrate the absorbing material This, in turn, is dependent on the force with which it is propelled and the density of the substance to be penetrated.

Figure 2.2   **The electromagnetic spectrum**

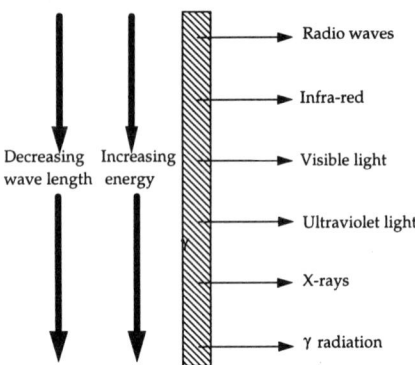

Ionising radiation can be classified into three categories each of which has a different power of penetration (Figure 2.3).

α particles produce intense ionisation but have poor penetration and a rapid loss of energy. These are relatively large and positively charged particles which can be stopped by a few centimetres of air or a few sheets of paper. For this reason, α radiation is not commonly used in therapy.

β particles result when a neutron within the nucleus disintegrates to form a proton and an electron. β particles are smaller and negatively charged and have a greater power of penetration than α particles; they can, however, be stopped by a few millimetres of material with the density of water or aluminium. Phosphorus-32 (^{32}P) and yttrium-90 (^{90}Y) are examples of those which may be used for therapeutic purposes; the patient's body provides an effective barrier against this type of radiation.

Figure 2.3   **Power of penetration of α, β and γ radiation**

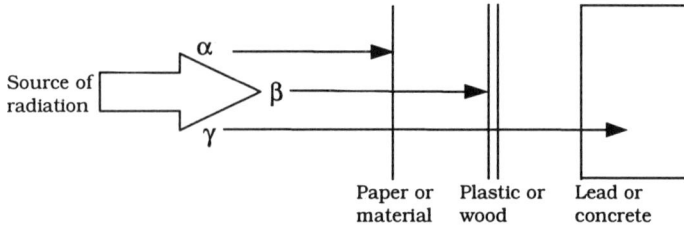

Gamma (γ) rays and X-rays are described as photons, discrete 'bundles' (quanta) of energy; this energy is transferred to the absorbing material liberating electrons, particularly those close to the nucleus, from their orbits causing ionisation. Ionisation can arise in several ways:

1. When a photon collides directly with an electron there is a transfer of energy to the electron; this ejects it from its orbit. Such a highly charged electron is capable of provoking further ionisation. This is described as the *Photoelectric Effect* (Figure 2.4a).

2. When a photon transfers only some of its energy to an escaping electron the photon is not absorbed but emerges as a photon of lower energy accompanying the electron. Both are capable of provoking further chemical interactions. This is termed the *Compton Effect* (Figure 2.4b).

3. Finally, high energy photons may interact directly with the nucleus producing two charged particles (positive and negative) capable of causing further ionisation. (Figure 2.4c).

Other particulate radiation may also be employed in the treatment of malignant disease. For example, protons (hydrogen nuclei) and deuterons (heavy hydrogen nuclei) are examples of positively charged particles used in radiation therapy. Negatively charged pi-mesons (pions), produced by high energy accelerators, can be used to invoke multiple atomic interactions whilst achieving deep penetration in the tissues.

Figure 2.4a   **The photoelectric effect**

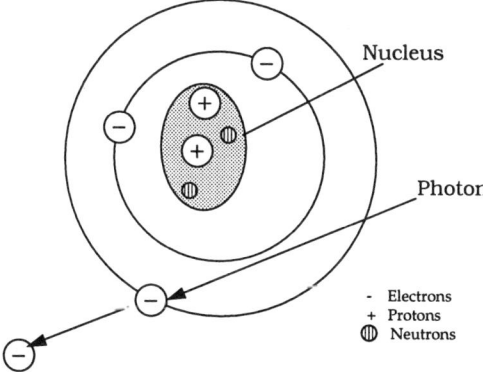

Nucleus

Photon

- Electrons
+ Protons
◐ Neutrons

Figure 2.4b **Compton scattering**

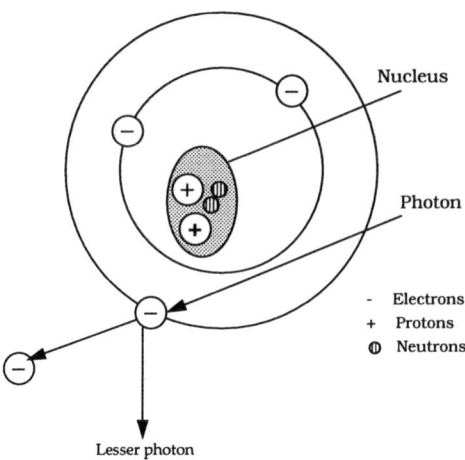

Nucleus

Photon

- Electrons
+ Protons
Ⓞ Neutrons

Lesser photon

Figure 2.4c **Production of an ion pair**

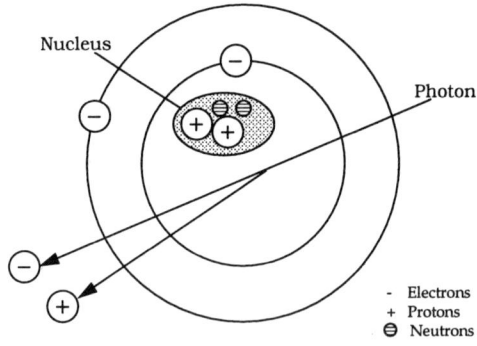

Nucleus

Photon

- Electrons
+ Protons
⊖ Neutrons

RADIATION ENERGY

Radiation energy is measured in *electron volts* (eV). One electronvolt represents the energy gained by an electron passing through an electrical potential of one volt (Martin and Harbison, 1996). However, since the electronvolt is a very small unit, radiation energy is usually described in kilo (1,000) or mega (1,000,000) electronvolts (keV or MeV).

With radiation energies less than 0.5MeV most interactions with atoms or molecules result from the photoelectric effect. At higher energies (i.e. between 0.5MeV and 5MeV) Compton scattering

14

predominates; the lesser (or scatter) photon may then interact with additional atoms through either Compton scattering or the photo-electric effect. Still higher energies result in the production of an electron and a positron from each photon of radiation (pair production). Positrons are positively-charged electrons that trigger a chain reaction eventually being annihilated by collision with ordinary negative electrons producing two photons of lesser energy. Such 'annihilation radiation' will then be absorbed through Compton scattering or the photoelectric effect.

The depth to which radiation can penetrate is a function of the energy with which it is propelled and the mass (weight) of the particle.

MEASUREMENT OF RADIATION

Administration of radiation as a therapeutic modality involves exposure of a tumour to a radioactive source. The ionising radiation thus passes through the exposed cells and tissues giving up energy to those cells; the dose of radiation received is measured in terms of the energy absorbed.

Radiation absorbed dose: the absorbed dose is a measure of the energy deposited by any form of ionising radiation. The unit of absorbed dose is the *gray* (Gy) (1Gy = 1Joule per kilogram). On occasions the dose administered is considerably less than 1Gy and then the units centigray (cGy) or milligray (mGy) are used; these are 100 centigray, 1000 milligray or 1 million microgray (μGy) in 1 Gray.

Dose equivalent: Although the absorbed dose would appear to be a useful concept allowing quantification of the radiation delivered, this is less useful in practice since the same dose of different types of radiation may produce different effects in biological systems (such as body tissues).

This difference in biological effectiveness must be taken into account when attempting to calculate the total biologically effective dose of radiation delivered (Martin and Harbison, 1986). To achieve this, the absorbed dose is multiplied by a quality factor (Q) which makes allowance for the relative effectiveness of the radiation involved. The result is known as the *dose equivalent*; the unit of measurement is the *sievert* (Sv). Again the dose equivalent may be considerably less than one sievert and smaller units are used. These are: millsieverts (10^{-3} sieverts) and microsieverts (10^{-6} sieverts) respectively (Table 2.2).

15

Table 2.2   **Radiation units**

Unit of absorbed dose	Gray (Gy)
Dose equivalent	Sieverts (Sv)
Specific activity	Becquerel (Bq)

The Becquerel measures the specific activity (rate of nuclear disintegration) of a radionuclide. Specifically, it measures the number of atoms of a particular radioisotope which disintegrate in one second. This is determined by the half life ($t_{1/2}$); knowledge of the specific activity is essential if precisely controlled doses of radiation are to be delivered. For any given source the specific activity gradually decreases at a rate determined by its half life.

RADIATION DETECTION

Since it is not possible to see, hear, smell, taste, touch or feel irradiation, specialised devices are required if it is to be detected. It is, therefore, essential that all staff involved wear a monitoring device (personal dosimeter) to monitor radiation exposure. Such devices are based on the physical or chemical effects of radiation.

The film badge is the most common personal dosimeter and comprises a piece of photographic film contained within a special holder. This is best worn at the site of maximum exposure, usually the abdomen. Care must be taken to ensure that the badge is not exposed to sources of heat or moisture as either of these may alter the validity of the film. Badges should be processed once a month since the accuracy of the film deteriorates after this period. The film is then compared to a film of known radiation exposure; this enables determination of the amount of radiation to which the wearer has been exposed. A careful record is kept of the total exposure of each individual since there are limits on the permissible occupational exposure to irradiation. The maximum permissible dose equivalent (for the whole body) is 50mSv per calendar year (The Ionising Radiations Regulations (IRR), 1985). The current regulations are summarised in Table 2.3.

Alternative detection devices may be used including the thermoluminescent dosimeter containing crystals which absorb radiation energy and, when heated, give off light measurement of which enables determination of the amount of radiation exposure. Although this is a sensitive device, it is expensive and does not

Table 2.3   **Ionising Radiations Regulations (1985): dose limits**

Dose limits	Employees >18yrs	Trainee <18yrs	Any other person
Whole body[1]	50mSv	15mSv	5mSv
Individual organs and tissue[1]	500mSv	150mSv	50mSv
Lens of the eye[2]	150mSv	45mSv	15mSv
Abdomen - women of reproductive capacity	13mSv in any 3 month period[3]		
Abdomen - pregnant women	10mSv during term of pregnancy[3]		

1. The above represent dose quantities from exposure to ionising radiation from external radiation together with the committed effective dose equivalent from radionuclides.

2. Represents the average dose equivalent from both external and internal radiation delivered between 2.5-3.5mm behind the surface of the eye.

3. Average exposure throughout abdomen

provide a permanent record of radiation exposure and, unlike the film badge, does not provide detailed information about the quality of the radiation to which the wearer has been exposed. Other personal dosimeters are available but they are not commonly used in current practice.

Those exposed to ionising radiation must understand that wearing a measurement device does *not* protect against radiation exposure but only provides a measure of the amount of radiation to which an individual has been exposed. For this reason, it is essential that it is realised that a monitoring device is unique to the individual and is not interchangeable. Such a device must be worn at all times when occupational exposure is likely.

The Geiger-Muller counter is a monitoring device used to measure the amount of radiation present in the environment (Figure 2.5). This consists, essentially, of a cylindrical metal tube filled with a suitable gas (e.g. argon) and sealed at one end by a thin window; a fine wire electrode runs through the middle. When atomic particles or radiation enter the tube, through the window, the gas ionises and

Figure 2.5   **Essential features of a Geiger-Muller counter**

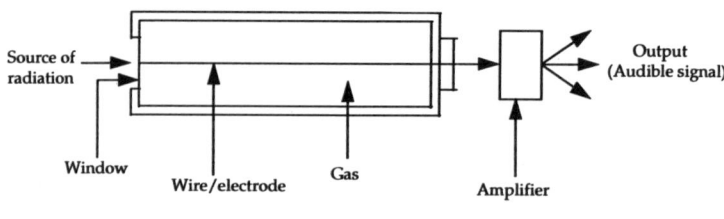

a current passes between the wall of the tube and the central electrode. This is detected by an attached recording device and gives a measure of both the amount and type of radiation present. Because radiation must pass through the window before it can be detected a Geiger-Muller counter is most suitable for high energy radiation.

In the hospital setting, a Geiger-Muller counter is used primarily when patients are treated by means of internal radiation therapy (brachytherapy). In this situation it is used at the bed side to determine if the source of radiation has been dislodged during treatment or to ensure that the source has been completely removed on completion of treatment.

A *Scintillation counter* works on a completely different principle and is intended to detect low energy radiation, such as α particles. In this case, radiation interacts with special chemicals (such as thallium-activated sodium iodide) causing them to emit light; it is detection of this light, converted into an electrical signal, which enables measurement of the amount of radiation present. These are primarily used in the laboratory setting.

RADIATION PROTECTION

Protection from radiation falls into two categories: protection for the population as a whole and protection for those likely to come into contact with higher doses of irradiation by nature of their work (occupational exposure).

The population is continuously exposed to radiation from naturally occurring sources such as cosmic rays, natural radioactive materials in rocks or soil and the small amounts of radioisotopes, primarily potassium, present in the human body. In addition, the increasing use of X-rays in diagnosis and as a therapeutic entity, combined with the small amount of radioactive fall-out from the testing of atomic weapons and from nuclear accidents, such as that in

Chernobyl (1986), will add to the natural radioactive load. It must, however, be recognised that the environmental hazard from the latter sources is small in comparison with that received from entirely natural sources.

The total annual dose of radiation from natural sources is approximately 1.25mSv and, in the average life time, approximately 90mSv. The dose received from natural sources is, however, difficult to calculate although, for the majority, this is very low; the population as a whole should receive no more than 50mSv per individual per annum.

When considering environmental exposure to radiation certain factors must be taken into account. These include:

- Length of time of exposure
- Total dose of radiation received
- Volume/area of the body exposed.

This can be represented by the simple formula:

$$\text{Biological effect} = \frac{\text{Dose x volume}}{\text{Time}}$$

The particular areas of concern are:

- Bone marrow - Due to the risk of myelosuppression and of carcinogenesis
- Gonads - Radiation may result in cessation of ovulation or spermatogenesis; the risk of genetic mutations in the ovum or sperm is increased.
- Lens of the eye - Conjunctivitis may be seen as an acute effect later followed by cataract development and corneal ulceration.

The extremities and skin can tolerate higher doses since they comprise primarily radioresistant tissues such as muscle, bone and tendons. The lethal dose of irradiation is approximately 4Sv; 50% of those receiving such a dose, over a short time period, will die, usually due to a secondary infection since immunocompetence is decreased as a result of bone marrow damage. When received over a period of years this dose is unlikely to cause death although health may be impaired.

Safety standards are laid down for the protection of radiological workers since some radiation exposure is often unavoidable for those involved in such work. Occupational exposure is currently limited to no more than 50mSv per year (IRR, 1985) for each year that the individual's age exceeds 18 years (Table 2.3). This means that the maximum dose equivalent should not exceed 50(N - 18) where N = the age in years.

As can be seen (Table 2.3) the current safety standards relating to permitted exposure are well below the 'danger level' and, in practice, they are seldom reached. It is likely that the regulations will be revised as a result of European legislation.

For the protection of those working with radiation, all radioactive materials *must* be shielded, both in storage and in use. Five-10cms of lead (or its equivalent) is needed to achieve effective shielding. This is thick enough to absorb all radioactive particles and most of the radiation (Aird and Williams, 1993).

Radioactive substances must be handled either by remote control or at a 'safe' distance since the intensity of radiation decreases by the square of the distance from the source of radiation (The Inverse Square Law) (Figure 2.6) (i.e. the further away the individual is from the source the smaller the dose of radiation to which he or she is exposed).

All equipment producing radiation (Ch 4) must be surrounded by thick walls or a maze which ensures that scattered radiation is kept within the machine room. When not in use the radioactive source is stored in a heavily screened unit and the machine cannot operate unless all doors and windows are closed. The efficiency of the machine, and the radiation scatter within the room, are regularly checked as is the level of radiation 'escaping' from the room.

All workers are legally required to wear a monitoring device which measures the amount of radiation to which they have been exposed; the dose received is calculated monthly and records are kept of the cumulative dose.

An individual who has received more than the permitted dose is immediately withdrawn from radiation work for a stipulated period, usually about 3 months. However, the risks to those abiding by the safety principles are slight.

Protection in the wards

Staff working in areas where radiation is employed must be familiar with radiation hazards and be able to minimise the risks in their daily practice. It must be recognised that patients undergoing external radiotherapy are not radioactive and, as such, pose no hazard to members of the caring team. Patients undergoing brachy-therapy, or receiving treatment with radioactive isotopes, are,

Figure 2.6   **The inverse square law**

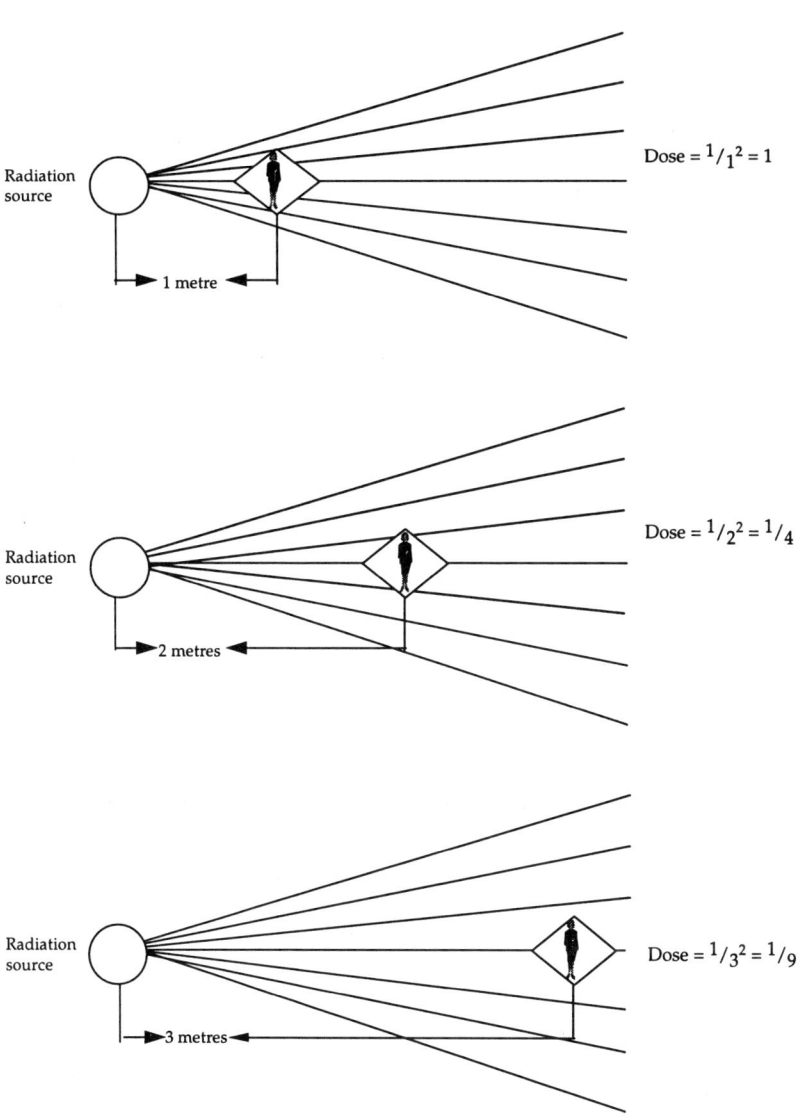

themselves, sources of radiation for as long as the treatment continues. Care of these patients is discussed in Ch 12.

In brief, the maximum dose rate at a distance of metre from each patient undergoing treatment must be calculated in order to determine times for safe working procedures and systems of work.

This is particularly important for nurses who must provide direct care for patients and also for porters who must regularly move patients around the hospital (Aird and Williams, 1993). The bed, or the door to the room, must bear a radioactive warning sign; the patient must not be allowed to leave either the room or the hospital whilst carrying the radioactive source and, to aid the protection of staff, should be encouraged to undertake as much of his/her care as possible. The time of exposure is calculated as if only one nurse were attending the patient. In fact, it is more appropriate for nursing duties to be shared so that individual exposure is reduced. It is, in any case, essential that the nurse spends only that time which is absolutely necessary at the bed side.

Additional protection must be available both for staff and for other patients. The need is assessed by the Radiation Protection Officer, a physicist who is responsible for safety in any unit where radiation is present. Ideally, patients are cared for in private rooms that are specifically designed for this purpose. Such rooms should be located in corners of the ward where only one wall connects with another room or a public thoroughfare (e.g. a corridor). In purpose-built units all walls will be lead-lined but, when such facilities are not available, mobile lead shields may be used at the bed side to provide additional protection. When appropriate shielding is available, patients undergoing brachytherapy may be nursed at the end of a general ward. Systemic radiotherapy treatment, using unsealed sources, means that the patient becomes radioactive so that this cannot be carried out unless appropriate facilities are available.

When brachytherapy is being undertaken the procedures and practices laid down for the safe custody of radioactive sources, and for the disposal of radioactive waste, must be strictly followed. Nurses must be informed about:

- The number and nature of the sources employed
- The total source strength
- The time and date of application
- The time and date of intended removal.

A lead container and long-handled forceps must be available in the unit at all times. A radioactive source must *never* be picked up with the hands; long-handled forceps, held as far from the body as possible, should be used to place dislodged or removed sources in the lead container prior to removal from the unit. If a source is lost, spilled or accidentally removed the radiation safety officer must be called and the following precautions taken:

1. Close all windows and, where appropriate, turn off air conditioners.
2. Clear all people from the room; the patient should be moved to another suitable room where radiation safety procedures are continued.
3. Drop absorbent material on to the spills; make no attempt to clean up the spillage.
4. Leave contaminated shoes in the room and close and lock the doors. The door may be sealed to prevent entry. The radiation physicist will determine the period for which the room must be sealed; this is dependent on the type and half life of the source. Once the room is declared safe it can be cleaned and re-used.
5. Contaminated individuals are restricted to a designated area where their clothes and body are surveyed (with a Geiger counter). Decontamination, if required, consists of multiple baths, cleansing especially the orifices, nail beds and body folds. Further action will be recommended by the physician if required.

When a source is lost all measures must be taken to find it; all linen must stay in the room and be monitored for radioactivity. The radiation safety officer must be notified. This is discussed further in Chapter 12.

REFERENCES

Aird EG, Williams JR, 1993, Brachytherapy. In: Williams JR, Thwaites DI (Editors), Radiotherapy Physics in Practice, Oxford Medical Publications, Oxford.

Leahy D, St Germain J, Varrichio C, 1979, The Nurse and Radiotherapy, C V Mosby, St Louis.

Martin A, Harbison SA, 1986, An Introduction to Radiation Protection (Third edition), Chapman and Hall, London.

Nias AHW, 1990, Radiation biology. In: Sikora K, Halnan KE (Editors), Treatment of Cancer (Second edition), Chapman and Hall Medical, London.

The Ionising Radiations Regulations, 1985. Her Majesty's Stationery Office, London, 1985, Schedule 1, pp 35-36.

CHAPTER 3   RADIOBIOLOGY

Radiobiology is the term used to describe the study of the effects of ionising radiation on the cells and tissues of living material such as the human body. The biological impact of radiation is primarily at the cellular level and varies between barely detectable damage to cell death. Its effects depend not only on the type of radiation but also on the number and types of cells affected. The extent of biological damage ultimately depends on the degree and permanence of the cell loss or damage and the type of functions compromised (Nias, 1990).

INTERACTIONS BETWEEN RADIATION AND CELLS

The basic difference between ionising radiations and the more commonly encountered, longer wavelength radiations, such as heat and light, is that the former have sufficient energy to cause ionisation (Martin and Harbison, 1986). The interactions between ionising radiation and body cells fall into four main categories: physical, physico-chemical, chemical and biological. It is these interactions that determine the cellular response either through a variety of mechanisms which may affect cell functions directly or indirectly. Cellular damage may affect both the construction and the function of the cell and, in the human body, are seen as clinical symptoms or side-effects.

As all cells are approximately 70% water, and water molecules are highly sensitive to ionisation, the effects of radiation can be demonstrated by considering its effects on water.

1. *Physical stage*: As radiation passes through a tissue some of its energy is transferred to that tissue causing ionisation (Ch 2) producing a variety of unstable, charged molecules. This reaction may be seen in water (H_2O):
$$H_2O \rightarrow H_2O^+ + e^-$$
Here H_2O^+ is a positive ion and e^- a negative ion.

2. *The physico-chemical stage*: These unstable and activated molecules (ions) subsequently undergo a variety of secondary reactions resulting in a number of new products some of which are stable molecules. It also causes the production of free radicals within the cell. For example, the positive ion dissociates (breaks down)
$$H_2O^+ \rightarrow H^+ + OH^\bullet$$

24

while the negative ion (e⁻) attaches to another available water molecule which then dissociates

$$H_2O + e^- \rightarrow H_2O^-$$
$$H_2O^- \rightarrow H^\bullet + OH^-$$

The products of these reactions are, therefore, the ions: H^+, OH^-, $H^\bullet$ and $OH^\bullet$. Both H^+ and OH^- are present in normal water and, although they have some potential for cellular damage through chemical reactions, they are more likely to recombine forming water (H_2O) and take no part in subsequent reactions.

The remaining products, $H^\bullet$ and $OH^{\bullet,}$ are free radicals (i.e. they have an unpaired electron) and are chemically extremely reactive. While they may recombine to form water, they are more likely to interact with other free radicals or with water or oxygen present in the cell causing further damage. Another reaction product is the strong oxidising agent hydrogen peroxide (H_2O_2) which is highly cytotoxic.

3. *Chemical stage*: Here the reaction products interact with important intracellular molecules. For example, both free radicals and oxidising agents, such as H_2O_2, may interact with DNA present in the cell nucleus disrupting chromosomal structure thus affecting the cell's reproductive ability.

4. *Biological stage*: It is the combined effects of the previous stages which result in biological damage. The time scale of such damage varies between a few minutes and many years depending on its nature. Damage can affect individual cells in various ways. For example, it may cause:

    a. The early death of the cell

    b. Inhibition or delay in mitosis

    c. A permanent modification which is passed on to the daughter cells.

Thus the effects of radiation on the human body are the result of damage to individual cells. These may be described as somatic - when they result from damage which affects only the irradiated person - and hereditary - when they affect the reproductive cells (gonads) and may be passed on to later generations.

THE CELL CYCLE

Both normal and cancer cells replicate in a similar fashion progressing through four distinct phases collectively known as the

Cell Cycle. These phases, diagrammatically represented in Figure 3.1, are G_1 - the post-mitotic gap, S - the synthetic phase, G_2 - the pre-mitotic gap and M - mitosis. G_1, the period following cell division, is a period of decreased metabolic activity when the cell carries out its designated physiological functions and when the proteins needed for maintenance of the cell are synthesised. Ribonucleic acid (RNA) and the other proteins needed for DNA synthesis are produced.

Some cells do not remain in active cycle but pass into a resting phase (G_0) when they become temporarily or permanently quiescent. This term can be applied to cells which will never divide (such as brain or neuronal cells) or others which are dormant but which are capable of being stimulated to re-enter the cell cycle when required (e.g. hepatocytes).

The onset of the S phase signals the end of G_2. During this phase DNA is synthesised and the chromosomal content of the cell is doubled.

During the pre-mitotic phase (G_2) the cell is prepared for division; protein and RNA are synthesised. Cells entering G_2 contain the duplicated genetic material synthesised during the S phase. Mitosis (the M phase) is the phase of the cycle in which the cell is physically dividing and reproducing two identical daughter cells.

Figure 3.1   **The cell cycle**

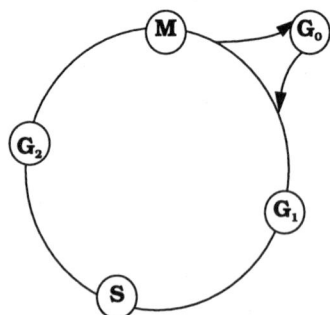

M = Mitotic phase. Cell divides to produce two identical daughter cells

G_0 = Resting phase. Cell is quiescent. All cell functions continue but cell is unable to divide

G_1 = Post-mitotic gap. A pre-synthetic phase in which the enzymes needed for DNA synthesis are produced

S = DNA synthesis takes place in preparation for cell division

G_2 = Pre-mitotic gap during which specialised proteins and RNA are synthesised in preparation for cell division.

Following mitosis, the two new cells either enter the cell cycle or pass into the resting phase (G_0).

The time interval between mitoses is called the *cell cycle time*. In general, the duration of M, S and G_2 are constant within any one cell type; the length of G_1 is, however, variable. As a result, the rate of replication varies amongst the different body tissues; this may also vary between normal and malignant cells. Normal cells with high growth fractions and short cell cycle times, such as the gastro-intestinal epithelium or the bone marrow, are particularly vulnerable to irradiation.

Cell replication is controlled by genetically determined stimuli which ensure that a new cell is produced only when an existing cell degenerates or dies. As a result, replication represents a fine balance between cellular reproduction and cell death. However, malignant cells differ from normal cells in several important ways. Although they divide at the same rate as the cells of their tissue of origin, cancer cells divide even in the absence of the internal signals induced by cell degeneration and/or death to the detriment of the host. Thus, at any given time, there will be a greater number of malignant cells in active replication.

However, like any other tissue, a tumour will contain a mixture of actively replicating cells, resting cells and permanently non-dividing cells. As the tumour mass increases, cells are gradually 'pushed' away from the blood supply and so receive an inadequate supply of oxygen and other nutrients, this leads to necrosis within the tumour. In general, these cells are of only limited concern for treatment purposes (see below).

RADIATION-INDUCED BIOLOGICAL EFFECTS

As we have seen, the effects of radiation at the cellular level may be direct or indirect (Travis, 1975; Withers and Peters, 1980; Hall and Cox, 1989). Target theory suggests that a direct 'hit' results when any of the key intracellular molecules are damaged (e.g. RNA and DNA).

Damage to DNA may cause:

1. Damage to or loss of, a base (thymine, adenine, cytosine or guanine)
2. Breakage of the hydrogen bond maintaining the DNA helix
3. Breakage of one or both chains in the DNA helix
4. Cross-linking between the chains of the DNA molecule after breakages.

Indirect effects occur when ionisation affects intracellular water causing damage as previously described.

Although a direct hit, and resulting damage to DNA and chromosomes, is the most effective and lethal injury caused by radiation, the large amount of intracellular water means that the likelihood of indirect effects due to ionisation of water is very much greater. Radiation can also affect other intracellular molecules, such as proteins, carbohydrates and enzymes. Such effects may potentiate radiation-induced damage within the cell.

Since all biochemical processes within the cell are controlled by DNA (Table 3.1) cells are most sensitive to radiation-induced damage during specific phases of the cell cycle when DNA synthesis may be disrupted or replication disturbed (Richter et al, 1985)

- In the M phase when the altered chromosomes lose their ability to produce two identical daughter cells.
- In the G_2 phase when protein synthesis is inhibited and changes occur in the chromosomes (DNA is the major component of chromosomes).

This means that the maximum effects of radiation occur just before and during the process of cell division. Cells are also vulnerable towards the end of G_1 when the substances needed for DNA synthesis are altered and, to a lesser extent, during the S phase when the intra-cellular DNA is doubled.

Table 3.1   **Functions of deoxyribonucleic acid (DNA)**

Control of all the biochemical processes of the cell
Promotion and maintenance of cellular function
Promotion and maintenance of cellular reproduction
i.e. Transfer of genetic information
     Cell reproduction
     Synthesis of proteins, enzymes and hormones

Radiation-induced damage may cause: faulty transcription of genetic information, defective repair, metabolic disturbances, accelerated ageing and mutation, all of which may affect a cell's ability to divide.

Changes in mitotic activity can be described as delayed-onset or complete inhibition. A delay in the onset of mitosis indicates that, although damage has occurred at some point during the cell cycle, intracellular repair has enabled division to take place.

Complete inhibition means that the cell is unable to divide; it may, however, continue to function. Thus, the lethal effects of radiation may not be apparent until the cell divides although, at times, five or six divisions may be required before cell death occurs.

Cellular damage is greatest in the presence of oxygen since this is necessary for the formation of some types of free radical so that, in hypoxic cells, the response to radiation is reduced. Certain drugs, such as metronidazole or misonidazole, may be used to increase sensitivity to radiation in hypoxic cells within a tumour. Such drugs are known as radiosensitisers (see p36).

OTHER FACTORS

The preceding discussion shows that the effects of radiation are not restricted to malignant cell populations. The ability of a cell or tissue to recover from such damage determines the ultimate biological impact.

Cell repair: In general, normal cells can repair partial damage whereas cancer cells lack this ability; rarely cancer cells may repair partial damage although this is a slow and inadequate process. Neither normal or malignant cells can repair total damage. Although the extent of damage increases with increasing radiation exposure it should be noted that fractionated exposure (see p43) does not, in general, reduce cell division to the same extent as the same dose given in a single exposure.

Repopulation: Repopulation of normal tissues following radiation-induced damage will permit such tissues to proliferate. Tumour cells are, in general, less likely to achieve this due to their inability to repair partial (or sub-lethal) damage.

Cells in the resting phase (G_0) may be recruited to replace cells lost through radiation-induced damage so that, during fractionated treatment, tumour cells may be redistributed. Thus spreading the dose over a prolonged period may reduce its biological impact (Parker, 1980).

However, ionising radiation may delay mitosis so that successive treatments may actually increase the number of cells in active replication thus increasing the effectiveness of subsequent doses. Normal cells are, as we have seen, more efficient than cancer cells in replacing those damaged by radiation and are much less likely to be delayed or redistributed in their cycle.

Not every cell within a tissue is lethally damaged or even affected by radiation so that, unless cell damage is extensive or if cells are not replaced quickly, only minimal effects may be seen on tissue function.

The vulnerability of a tissue to the lethal effects of radiation, therefore, depends on the responsiveness of the cells and their ability to repair the injuries sustained (Parker, 1980). Repopulation of normal tissues following radiation-induced damage will permit such tissues to proliferate.

CELL SURVIVAL CURVES

Radiobiological effects are often quoted in terms of the cell survival curve (Figure 3.2). This is obtained by plotting the fraction of a cell population which survives against the dose of radiation received. The resultant curve is almost exponential (i.e. the higher the dose, the lower the survival). The dose required to reduce the number of cells in any given population to 37% of the original number is described as D_{37} (Lowry, 1974). This is used to describe a survival curve and, as such, can be used as an index of radiosensitivity (see below).

However, if the curve is plotted with the surviving fraction on a logarithmic scale (Figure 3.2) the curve becomes a straight line that is easier to interpret. But, in practice, the logarithmic 'curve' does not form an exactly straight line since there is a small 'shoulder' to overcome before the curve is exponential. This can be measured on the vertical axis by extrapolation giving the value of N. This provides a measure of a different parameter of radiosensitivity, threshold resistance (i.e. the initial resistance to the effects of radiation). The term D_0 represents the truly exponential portion of the curve and is the term more commonly used.

RADIOSENSITIVITY

As has been shown, cells that are exposed to radiation are likely to undergo a sequence of changes which ultimately result in biological damage. Radiosensitivity is the term used to describe the degree and speed of the response to radiation of a given tissue (normal or malignant).

Those cells which replicate frequently (i.e. have a short cell cycle time) appear to be most sensitive to radiation as they exhibit signs of damage more rapidly than those with a longer cell cycle time or than resting cells. However, it is not entirely clear whether such cells are

Figure 3.2a   **The cell survival curve**

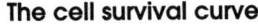

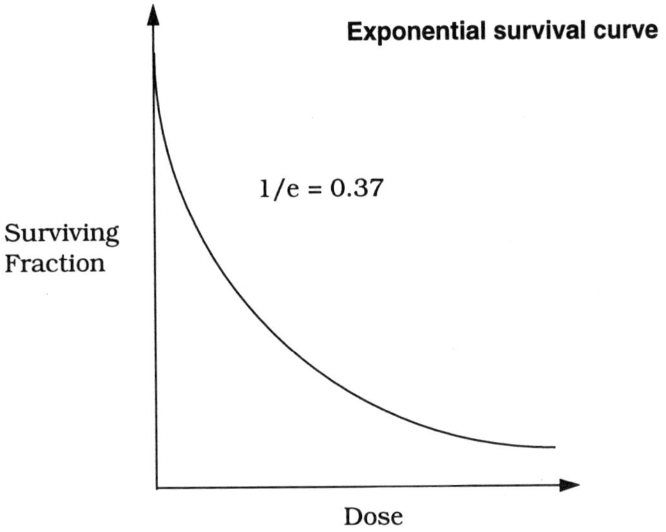

Exponential survival curve

$1/e = 0.37$

Surviving
Fraction

Dose

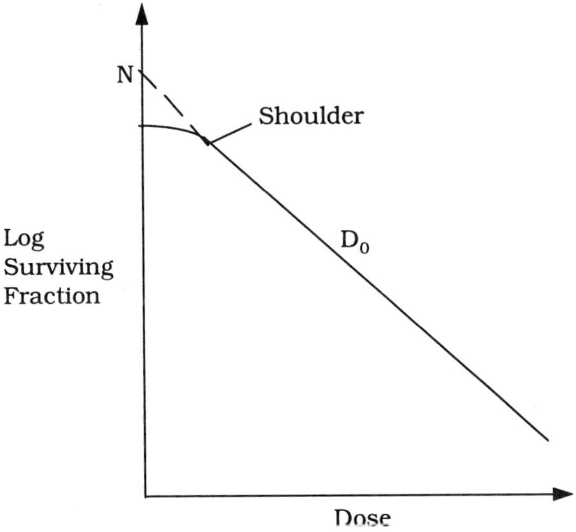

N

Shoulder

Log
Surviving
Fraction

D_0

Dose

e is the mathematical term used to represent the exponential constant
and = 2.718. $1/e = 0.37$ which is equivalent to 37%

are truly more sensitive to radiation or whether, due to rapid replication, cell loss is manifested more quickly. However, as has been shown, radiosensitivity also varies within the cell cycle with cells being most vulnerable at or close to mitosis (i.e. the latter stages of G and during G_2; resistance is greatest during the S phase (Hall, 1978)). Radiosensitivity does not, however, equate with the curability of a tumour at a specific site. Radiosensitivity within malignant tissues varies not only with the type of tumour but also with its size and location.

Some of the most radiosensitive tumours are also those which are the most anaplastic and undifferentiated, and thus metastasise both early and rapidly, so that they cannot be cured by radiotherapy. Thus, for clinical purposes, a tumour is termed radiosensitive when it can be eradicated by a dose of radiation that permits recovery of normal cells included in the treatment field.

Almost all cancer cells can be destroyed by radiation although, at times, the dose required is so high that normal cells are also irreversibly damaged; such tissues are described as radioresistant.

Normal tissues can also be classified according to their degree of radiosensitivity. Tissues described as radiosensitive include:

- Bone marrow
- Gastrointestinal epithelium
- Genito-urinary tract
- Gonads
- Lymphoid tissue
- Hair follicles.

Organs and tissues described as having a low degree of radio-sensitivity include mature bone and cartilage, the thyroid gland, the brain and spinal cord and the liver.

Oxygenation

As previously discussed the level of oxygenation can enhance the effects of radiation. This can be affected by a variety of anatomical and physiological factors which affect the blood supply; this can, in turn, alter tissue concentrations of oxygen.

EFFECTS OF RADIATION ON TISSUES

When a tissue is exposed to radiation the effects may be dramatic particularly if its cells are destroyed. When cell function declines and degeneration becomes apparent, the release of toxic waste products results in an inflammatory response in affected tissues causing oedema which increases as cellular destruction increases. Remaining cells may slough off tissue surfaces so that the tissue becomes denuded and may become ulcerated resulting in symptoms such as mucositis and stomatitis, nausea and vomiting, cystitis or diarrhoea.

Death occurs in similar ways in both normal and malignant cells:

- Death may be *immediate* due to irreversible damage to DNA; cells die before they reach the next mitosis, usually within 2 hours of exposure. This mechanism is responsible for the immediate side-effects of radiation. Such damage is uncommon at the sort of doses commonly used in therapy although a few cell types, which do not normally go through a reproductive cycle (e.g. small lymphocytes) appear to be very sensitive to this type of damage (Nias, 1990).

- Death may be *delayed* after mutation of DNA. Limited functions usually continue until the M phase when the cell is unable to divide (mitotic death). This may occur within 24 hours or be delayed for prolonged periods depending on the generation time of affected cells. This is responsible for the long-term effects of radiation.

- Radiation exposure can result in the formation of giant or sterile cells which show no loss of functional integrity but which cannot divide. These degenerate slowly dying a 'natural' death.

Normal cells begin to repair radiation-induced damage within a few hours of exposure although, following irradiation, a tissue may not regain its full pre-treatment function due to the presence of fibrosis or the formation of scar tissue; atrophy and/or necrosis may follow destruction of capillaries within affected tissues. The responses observed are dependent upon the degree of damage incurred.

Cells and tissues dividing slowly (e.g. neuronal cells or muscle) show a less dramatic response to radiation since only few cells are in active replication at any given time. However, although cellular destruction is limited, damage to the capillaries is likely and may result in fibrosis, atrophy or necrosis in affected tissues. Normal tissues, however, may be partly protected from radiation by inducing anoxia. Local anoxia can be achieved by use of tourniquet or by induction of hypothermia.

THERAPEUTIC EXPOSURE TO RADIATION

It is clear that exposure to ionising radiation can be very damaging to body cells and tissues. This can be used to good effect in treating malignant disease when radiotherapy can be employed to cause destruction of the tumour. However, despite the many precautions, some degree of damage to normal tissues is inevitable although it must be remembered that this occurs only when these are included in the treatment field.

Normal tissue responses are usually referred to as the side-effects of radiotherapy. Radiation-induced side-effects are, therefore, usually localised and located within the treatment field although they may be generalised when they are often described as 'radiation sickness' or 'radiation syndrome' (see Ch 6).

Tissue responses are described in terms of three general categories

- *Acute side-effects* occur during, or shortly after, treatment as the result of immediate responses to radiation. They are primarily related to the total dose and the degree of fractionation (see p43) and often increased in areas of rapid cell turn-over such as the skin, gastrointestinal tract and bone marrow. The effects are usually self limiting subsiding once treatment ceases.

- *Sub-acute side-effects* occur weeks or months after treatment and are usually related to the total therapeutic dose, particularly in tissues with a slow rate of cell turnover (e.g. epithelial tissues) so that damage may not occur until months after radiation. Due to the time delay, such damage can be difficult to differentiate from progression of disease. Prompt recognition allows rapid treatment and prevents serious complications.

- *Late/chronic responses*, related to the total therapeutic dose received by particularly radiosensitive tissues, may arise between 1 and 5 years (or longer) after exposure. Cellular alterations may not be seen for considerable periods due to slow cellular proliferation and, unlike acute reactions, are not always amenable to treatment. Effects include tissue necrosis, fistulae and dense fibrosis. They may be related to previous acute or sub-acute side-effects. Carcinogenesis is another potential complication that is not seen for many years after exposure.

MODIFIERS OF THE EFFECTS OF RADIATION

Since the aim of radiotherapy is to cause maximum damage to malignant cells while minimising that to normal tissues considerable research has been devoted to attempts to improve the therapeutic ratio (e.g. Hellman, 1985; Wasserman and Kligerman, 1987). For example, combined approaches to therapy, using both chemotherapy and radiotherapy, may enhance tumour cell kill. Chemotherapeutic agents such as bleomycin, doxorubicin, cisplatin, cyclophosphamide, and actinomycin-D are often used alongside radiation to take advantage of their synergistic effects and achieve greater cell kill than could be achieved by either therapy if it were used independently (Hilderley, 1992).

Radiosensitisers: Radiosensitisers are chemical compounds which are used to potentiate or enhance the effect of radiation on cells or tissues (Phillips, 1977; 1981). The rationale underlying this approach is the knowledge that the presence of oxygen enhances the damaging effects of radiation and that many tumours have hypoxic portions that are radioresistant (Hilderley and Dow, 1991).

Chemical radiosensitisers are agents which replace oxygen in hypoxic cells thus enhancing radiation effectiveness. They appear to act by promoting fixation of the free radials (e.g. OH• generated by radiation-induced damage) thus preventing intracellular repair. Compounds in current use include metronidazole and misonidazole. Pyrimidine analogues have also be found to be useful radiosensitisers as they are readily incorporated into DNA thus inhibiting repair of sublethal damage (Phillips, 1981; Fowler, 1985; Hellman, 1985).

Another group of compounds which has been shown to have radio-sensitising effects is the perfluorocarbons which absorb large amounts of oxygen when exposed to hyperbaric conditions releasing this when environmental oxygen is reduced. Such compounds, therefore, serve to transport oxygen to hypoxic areas and, again enhance the effect of radiation.

Radioprotectors: The need to protect normal cells from radiation-induced damage is a continuing challenge in radiotherapy since agents employed must be selective to healthy tissues if the desired results are to be achieved. This approach is, therefore, directed towards increasing the therapeutic ratio thus enabling damaged cells to repair radiation-induced damage. This is achieved by capturing free electrons so that they can participate in no further chemical reactions.

Sulphydryl compounds are the most commonly investigated radio-protective agents. These enable repair to take place through the chemical process of reduction when repair of critical molecules, damaged by ionisation, is aided by donation of a hydrogen atom from the sulphydryl group. Such agents have been described as 'scavengers' in their affinity for the products of irradiated water (Wasserman and Kligerman, 1987).

IMPLICATIONS FOR HEALTH CARE PROVIDERS

Any situation in which therapies are combined to promote enhanced cytotoxicity may result in an accompanying increase in the incidence of side-effects and a decrease in patient comfort. Radiosensitisers, for example, have their own specific toxic effects which include neuro-toxicity and central nervous system symptoms such as confusion, somnolence and transient coma. Nausea and vomiting may also occur; these effects seem to be dose-related (Noll, 1990).

Patients must be informed of the likelihood of such effects as their occurrence may be frightening to these vulnerable individuals. Supportive care must be provided. Since many of these approaches are currently under investigation it is also important to ensure that the occurrence of side-effects is closely monitored and documented.

REFERENCES

Fowler JF, 1985, Chemical modifiers of radiosensitivity - theory and reality. A review, International Journal of Radiation Oncology, Biology and Physics, **11**, 665-674.

Hall E, 1978, Radiobiology for the Radiologist (Second edition), Harper and Row, Philadelphia.

Hall EJ, Cox JD, 1989, Physical and biologic basis of radiation therapy. In: Moss WT, Cox JD (Editors), Radiation Oncology: Rationale, Techniques, Results, CV Mosby, St Louis

Hellman S, 1985, Principles of radiation therapy. In: DeVita VT, Hellman S, Rosenberg SA (Editors), Principles and Practice of Oncology, Volume 1 (Second edition), JB Lippincott, Philadelphia.

Hilderley LJ, 1992. Radiotherapy. In: Groenwald SL, Frogge MH, Goodman M, Yarbro CH, (Editors), Treatment Modalities. Part III from Cancer Nursing Principles and Practice (Second edition), Jones and Bartlett Publishers, Boston.

Hilderley LJ, Dow KH, 1991, Radiation oncology. In: Baird SB,

McCorkle R, Grant M (Editors), Cancer Nursing: A Comprehensive Textbook, WB Saunders Co, London.

Lowry S, 1974, Fundamentals of Radiation Therapy, English Universities Press Ltd., London.

Martin A, Harbison SA, 1986, An Introduction to Radiation Protection (Third edition), Chapman and Hall, London.

Nias AHW, 1990, An Introduction to Radiobiology, John Wiley and Sons, Chichester.

Noll L, 1990, Chemical modifiers of radiation therapy. In: Hassey K, Hilderley L (Editors), Nursing Perspectives in Radiation Oncology, Delmar Publishers, New York.

Parker R, 1980, Principles of radiation oncology. In: Haskell C, (Editor), Cancer Treatment, WB Saunders Co., Philadelphia.

Phillips TL, 1977, Chemical modification of radiation effect, Cancer, **39**, 987-999.

Phillips TL, 1981, Sensitisers and protectors, Seminars in Oncology, **8**, 65-82.

Richter MP, Share FS, Goodman RL, 1985, Principles of radiation therapy. In: Calabrese P, Schein PS, Rosenberg SA (Editors), Medical Oncology: Basic Principles and Clinical Management of Cancer, MacMillan, New York.

Travis E, 1975, Primer of Medical Radiobiology, Year Book Medical Publisher, Chicago.

Wasserman TH, Kligerman M, 1987, Chemical modifiers of radiation effect. In: Perez CA, Brady LW (Editors), Principles and Practice of Radiation Oncology, JB Lippincott, Philadelphia.

Withers HR, Peters LJ, 1980, Biologic aspects of radiotherapy. In: Fletcher GH (Editor), Textbook of Radiotherapy (Third edition), Lea and Febiger, Philadelphia.

CHAPTER 4   USE OF RADIATION TO TREAT CANCER

As previously described, the biological impact of radiation is primarily at the cellular level where the damage can be so slight as to be barely detectable or severe and cause cell death. It is the latter effects that are exploited in cancer treatment when radiation may be used with curative or palliative intent. As a result, the aims and objectives of cancer treatment must be clearly defined before the method of treatment is selected for individual patients.

Although all types of living cell can be destroyed by ionising radiation the dose required to achieve a particular level of cell destruction is extremely variable. In addition, since tumours are sited in, or on, tissues whose function must be maintained, and are surrounded by healthy structures, the effects of radiation are not restricted to malignant cells; tumours cannot be treated in isolation. Thus, the aim of radiotherapy is to deliver the highest possible dose of radiation to cancer-bearing tissues while limiting the risk of damage to surrounding normal tissues to an acceptable level. In some cancers, such as that of the stomach, these aims are, however, incompatible since the radiosensitivity of adjacent tissues exceeds that of the cancer (Williams and Thwaites, 1993). In general, however, the larger the tumour volume the lower the dose of radiation that can be given safely without exceeding the tolerance of associated normal tissue (Nias, 1990). The radiotherapeutic aims of palliative treatment may be more limited (see below).

Since radiotherapy is not without side-effects the risks and the benefits (e.g. the likelihood of cure or control) must be carefully evaluated. Once radiation is selected, the source and technique best suited to the objectives of treatment are identified taking into account the many variables influencing the success or failure of such treatment. The method of treatment is largely determined by the site, type and stage of the tumour; the other factors influencing the choice are discussed later in this chapter.

CURATIVE TREATMENT

Clearly, the primary objective of curative radiation is eradication of the disease. Effective treatment will mean that neither the disease nor its treatment will markedly affect the life span. However, when discussing malignant disease, the concept of cure is a difficult one since malignant cells may be present even though they cannot be detected by current diagnostic techniques. The term for this situation, when the patient shows no evidence of cancer but is not necessarily cancer-free, is complete remission. The term 5-year disease-free survival is also frequently used. Since metastasis or recurrence is most likely during the first 5 years following diagnosis and treatment, the patient is regarded to be cured if he experiences a 5-year disease-free period following treatment. However, although for some tumours this time period is appropriate, for others it is too long or too short.

For tumours with a rapid mitotic rate a one or two year disease-free period is regarded as curative whereas, for those with dividing more slowly, 15-20 disease-free years may be needed before the treatment can be considered successful. Biological cure refers to a patient having no evidence of disease, who has the same life expectancy as person who has never had cancer and who ultimately dies of unrelated causes (van Eys, 1987).

In general, tumours which are curable by radiotherapy are those which are radiosensitive and relatively localised; anaplastic cells are usually more responsive to radiation than those which are well-differentiated. A high growth fraction (high percentage of cells in active division) also increases the vulnerability to irradiation.

The location of a tumour, and the extent of metastasis, must be also be determined since the presence of distant metastases usually limits the value of radiotherapy as a curative option. It may then be used in conjunction with chemotherapy when it may have a separate, additive or interactive effect. Alternatively, radiotherapy may be used in conjunction with surgery, either pre- or post-operatively, when it may enhance the chance of cure or control.

Pre-operatively radiotherapy can be used to decrease the size of a tumour and, perhaps, to avoid the need for mutilative surgery. It may also decrease the risk of tumour spread (seeding) following surgical intervention. A lag period is usually left between radiotherapy and surgery so as to decrease the risk of complications due to the acute side-effects of radiotherapy, and to permit recovery of normal tissues before surgery is undertaken; ideally this time interval is not so long as to permit regrowth of the tumour. The length of this lag phase is variable and does not usually exceed 3 months; it is dependent on the type, site and total dose of radiation as well as the area of the treatment field (Parker, 1980).

Use of radiation to treat cancer

Post-operative radiotherapy can be directed towards eradicating residual, although undetected, malignant cells thus decreasing the risk of recurrence; alternatively, unresectable lymph nodes may be irradiated. Again there may be a time lag between the two therapies to allow complete wound healing before radiotherapy is initiated.

PALLIATIVE TREATMENT

Some types of cancer are not amenable to cure by radiotherapy; others may present at a stage when cure is no longer possible. Under such conditions, radiation can be used for palliation of specific distressing symptoms and can significantly improve the quality of the patient's life. Indications for palliative radiotherapy include pain, compression of vital structures such as the brain, spinal cord or superior vena cava, malignant effusions that are causing distress, pain or dyspnoea, haemorrhage or the presence of bony metastases that are likely to cause a pathological fracture, particularly if these are present in weight-bearing bones such as the femur. When caring for such patients it is important to remember that the aim of palliative therapy is to achieve palliation of a symptom(s) so that the dose employed is only as high as is necessary to symptom relief; palliative therapy which results in serious or acute side-effects, thus creating further distress, is regarded as bad palliative therapy. This is discussed in greater depth in Ch 13.

THE TREATMENT PLAN

Before radiotherapy commences, extensive diagnostic testing and staging procedures are undertaken to define the treatment field, ensure the accuracy of daily treatment and protect surrounding tissues from radiation-induced damage. Treatment planning is the process through which the necessary treatment is established. Its aims are:

1. To localise the tumour volume and to establish the total volume of tissue to be irradiated.
2. To calculate the total dose of radiation necessary and, by placing the tumour in its anatomical context, identify any constraints to administration of the desired dose.
3. To determine the optimum treatment configuration needed to irradiate the target volume to the prescribed dose within the clinical constraints particular to individual patients.
4. To establish the dose distribution in the patient.

5. To prepare clear and unambiguous instructions for the therapeutic radiographers concerning the treatment of individual tumours and/or patients   (Redpath et al, 1993).

A radiotherapy simulator is   used to produce an image of the treatment field. This is similar to the treatment machine thus enabling a reproducible plan to be achieved. In other words, it simulates treatment so that consistent and accurate treatment can be ensured. During simulation, the target volume is defined and localised   using X-rays, scans and physical landmarks. The patient must be positioned exactly as he will be during his forthcoming therapy. Immobilisation may be necessary. Devices, such as head-restraints or plaster casts, may be required to ensure accurate positioning. Such devices not only help to maintain the patient's position but may also promote comfort and provide support.

Once the radiation field has been determined, this is carefully marked on to the patient's skin using either ink or small tattoos to identify the co-ordinate points of the treatment field as a guide to correct positioning during therapy.

The couch used for the simulator must be identical to that used for the treatment unit, usually flat-topped and hard. It must be iso-centrically mounted so that it rotates around the isocentre and it must also be able to move vertically, laterally and longitudinally through the isocentre (see p45). Computerised axial tomography (CAT scan), magnetic resonance imaging (MRI) and ultrasound can also be used as aids in locating the tumour more precisely providing clear anatomic guidelines. This is particularly important when the tumour is difficult to image conventionally or when a detailed image of the surrounding soft tissues is required.

Such techniques provide not only verification of the tumour but also indicate its relationship to vital structures and its depth in the tissues thus providing an accurate cross-sectional outline which, in turn, helps to delineate the depth and volume of tissue to be treated. This is essential if an accurate treatment plan is to be defined.

An anatomical outline of the patient is made and the position of the tumour is marked as accurately as possible. Isodose curves are then constructed and an optimum treatment plan is designed. Iso-dose curves represent the percentage of radiation remaining in a beam at given depths of normal tissues and enable accurate calculation of the dose of radiation as it passes through a tissue to be established (Figure 4.1).

Figure 4.1   **An isodose curve**

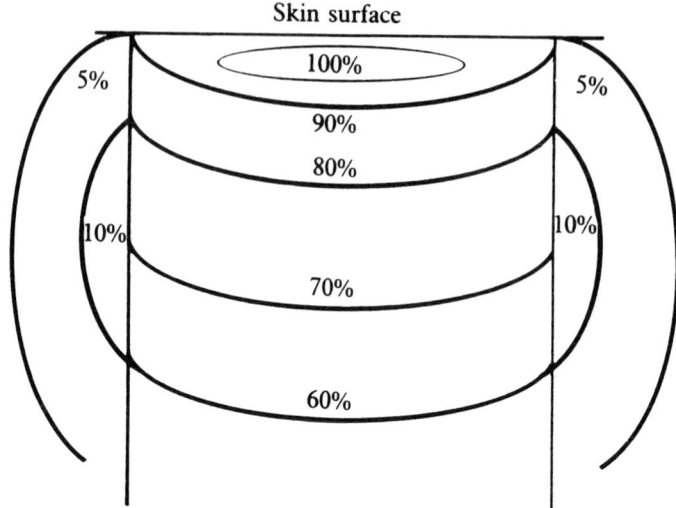

The treatment plan is the result of adding together the isodose curves of all the radiation fields to be used in treating individual tumours. This should produce an even dose of radiation across the tumour volume with less than a 5% variation. The dose to surrounding tissues, particularly those which are radiosensitive, should be as small as possible.

The success of radiation therapy depends on the interactions between many factors related both to the tumour itself and to the patient to be treated. The aim is to produce the maximum effect on the tumour while causing minimum damage to adjacent normal cells. It is achieved by considering the dose:time relationship, the volume of tissue to be irradiated and the general condition of the patient.

Dose of radiation: This is determined by the radiosensitivity of the tumour, the therapeutic ratio and the patient's condition. Radiation is capable of destroying virtually all cancer cells although the dose need may be such as to cause irreversible damage to normal cells included in the treatment field; such tumours are regarded as being radioresistant. Radiosensitivity, on the other hand, permits a tumour to be eradicated by a dose of irradiation which allows the recovery of normal cells. Radiosensitivity is usually commensurate with that of the tissue of origin and, as generation times vary between different cell types, some cells are more vulnerable to radiation than others.

Cells that are rapidly dividing (e.g. bone marrow, gastrointestinal epithelium) are more sensitive than those dividing slowly thus, the greater the number of cells in active replication, the greater the cytotoxic effect. This, combined with the fact that poorly differentiated and immature cells are particularly radiosensitive, is used to good effect when the tumour lethal dose is calculated.

Sensitivity is also dependent on the presence of oxygen; killing hypoxic cells requires a dose of radiation two to three times higher than that needed to achieve the same effect in well-oxygenated cells. It is, therefore, common to deliver the total dose in daily fractions so that, as each fraction is delivered, tumour shrinkage brings previously hypoxic cells closer to the blood supply enhancing the effects of successive treatments. Fractionation also prevents the acute radiation exposure which is likely if the total dose is delivered in a single treatment.

The radiosensitivity of a tumour is, therefore, determined by:

- The rate of replication (cell division) in the tissue of origin
- The degree of differentiation
- The size, location and extent
- The degree of oxygenation (dependent on the blood supply).

Calculation of the tumour lethal dose (TLD) takes the radio-sensitivity of a tumour into account. This is the dose which has a 95% probability of control or cure.

The second factor that is taken into account when calculating the radiation dose is the therapeutic ratio (TR). This represents the relationship between the dose of radiation which can be tolerated by the normal tissues adjacent to the tumour and that required to destroy malignant cells; this is represented by the equation:

$$\text{Therapeutic ratio} = \frac{\text{Normal tissue tolerance dose}}{\text{Tumour lethal dose}}$$

Normal tissue tolerance is calculated by comparison with a known (standard) dose to which a test population developed a severe complication rate within 5 years of treatment. The maximal tolerance dose is that which results in a 50% complication rate; the minimal tolerance dose is that producing a 5% severe complication rate.

A TR below 1 means that radiotherapy cannot be used to treat a tumour without extensive damage to surrounding normal tissues; a TR in excess of 1 means that it is likely that the tumour can be successfully treated by means of irradiation.

Use of radiation to treat cancer

The dose:time relationship: As previously stated, administration of the tumour lethal dose as a single treatment could result in acute radiation exposure which would be extremely detrimental to health thus defeating the objective. Thus the total dose is divided into smaller doses (fractions) which are usually given on a daily basis, so that exposure is protracted. Although there may be some variation due to local policy, fractionated doses are usually delivered on 5 days per week over a period ranging from 2-8 weeks; this ensures a 2 day rest period in every week. However, although five treatments a week for six weeks has been shown to be a clinically acceptable regime, Nias (1990) suggests that this approach is based more on expediency than upon radiobiological principles. A single regime of fractionation cannot possibly be appropriate for every tumour (Williams and Thwaites, 1993).

The practice of fractionation was introduced in an attempt to irradiate as many tumour cells as possible during mitosis and to make use of the four 'R's' of radiobiology:

- Recovery of cells from radiation-induced damage
- Repopulation of both the tumour and normal cells between fractions
- Re-oxygenation of the tumour during the course of therapy
- Redistribution of normal and tumour cells in the cell cycle.

Since the immediate effects of irradiation occur within the first two hours of exposure this approach allows both normal and cancer cells to attempt repair between successive treatments. As normal cells are better able to achieve repair, and to achieve this both more rapidly and more effectively, fractionation may also help to minimise the damage to normal tissues; it may also enhance the effect of radiotherapy since, as previously discussed, it will increase the number of well-oxygenated cells within the tumour. In general, however, an extension of the overall time over which the total dose is delivered will reduce its biological effectiveness (Easson and Pointon, 1985; Nias, 1990). If a dose is omitted, for whatever reason, an extra treatment may be added; alternatively, the daily fraction may be increased.

In practice there is considerable variation in fractionation regimes. Within the UK these may range from 30 fractions for 5 days a week over 6 weeks to 6 fractions delivered twice a week over 3 weeks. It has yet to be proved that any particular regime is optimally effective in treating specific tumours or with respect to local tumour control or radiation-induced morbidity. Accelerated fractionation regimes may be used in which the usual number of fractions is given over a shorter period of time often involving administration of more than one daily fraction (Nias, 1990). One example is the CHART regime (continuous hyperfractionated accelerated radiation treatment) which comprises 36 fractions of 1.4Gy, given three times daily at 6 hour intervals, over 12 days including the weekend (Saunders and Dische, 1986). However, while such a regime may reduce the extent of re-population by tumour cells, the time interval may be too short to permit re-oxygenation within the tumour between fractions. Using this approach, treatment is completed before the radiation reaction starts; normal tissues can then recover without further radiation-induced damage (Hall, 1993).

The volume of the treatment field: The clinical response to radio-therapy is influenced by the volume of both tumour and normal tissues included in the treatment field. As the volume of the tumour increases so too does the dose of radiation needed to ensure that the probability of cure or control is increased. This is, of necessity, associated with an increase in the volume of normal tissue included within the treatment field which may restrict the total dose of radiation that can be tolerated if it is not to cause an unacceptable increase in morbidity. The cure rate that can be achieved with radio-therapy is always limited by the dose that can be tolerated by adjacent normal tissues. Thus care is taken to keep the total volume exposed to radiation as small as possible so that it includes only the tumour and the smallest possible amount of normal tissue.

Radiation beams may be directed in a number of different directions so as to deliver the appropriate dose to the tumour whilst 'sparing' normal tissue. Since single-field treatments are generally used only for palliative purposes multiple beams are commonly used in the treatment of any tumour. By placing the patient in different positions on the treatment couch the use of appropriate beam directions can be maximised. When this approach is taken the radiation dose is calculated at the point at which absorption of radiation reaches its maximum intensity (Dietz, 1979).

Alternatively, rotation therapy may be employed when the source of radiation is rotated around the patient so that the geometric centre of the target volume (i.e. the tumour) is at the centre of the rotation (the isocentre). Wedge filters may be used to maintain a uniform dosage over the target volume (Easson and Pointon, 1985).

In general, if the volume of tissue to be treated is small, the total dose can be increased and the side-effects are likely to be less severe. When large volumes of tissue are to be irradiated it is necessary to protract treatment over an extended period.

The general condition of the patient: There is no doubt that the patient's general condition may significantly affect his response to radiotherapy as well as the incidence of side-effects. A patient who is depressed, nutritionally depleted and generally unwell is unlikely to withstand the rigours of his treatment as well as a patient who is both physically and emotionally well.

Although external beam therapy is less influenced by the patient's general condition than is, for example, surgery it may not be appropriate for the patient who is already severely compromised, particularly if there is little likelihood of cure or control. The frequency and duration of treatment may result in considerable disruption to the usual pattern of activity and the side-effects may exacerbate pre-existing physical and/or emotional problems. Even after treatment is complete, and cure has been achieved, patients may experience irreversible changes affecting either their functional ability, their appearance or their mental state.

Health care practitioners have an important role to play in preparing the patient for radiotherapy. Realistic presentation of the aims of treatment and potential side-effects will increase his understanding and enable him to become an active participant in his treatment and care.

EXTERNAL BEAM THERAPY (teletherapy)

External beam therapy is the most common form of radiotherapy and is normally performed with photon beams, generally high energy X-rays produced by a linear acceleration but gamma (γ) ray beams and lower energy X-rays may also be used. Although therapy with electrons is widely used, treatment with other particle radiations has also been proposed and, in some cases (e.g. neutron therapy) extensively tested. However, it now appears that neutrons offer no therapeutic benefit (Williams and Thwaites, 1993) although some charged particle beams (e.g. pions or protons) may offer some clinical advantages.

Different types of equipment are used to generate ionising radiation for the external treatment of various tumours. Kilovoltage equipment has been extensively used in cancer therapy and is widely discussed in the literature. In recent years, however, its use has diminished as megavoltage therapy and electrons have replaced it in most clinical applications. Kilovoltage therapy does, however, still have a role to play in the range of therapies available for treating malignant disease (Klevenhagen and Thwaites, 1993). Its main advantage is that of relatively low cost when compared with that of megavoltage therapy.

Radiation machines, similar to those used in X-ray diagnosis, are used to generate low level energy, ranging from 40-140keV, and are used to treat superficial lesions (i.e. those no deeper than 1cm). At this voltage, radiation particles can penetrate only short distances before their energy is released and absorbed. The maximum radiation dose is, therefore, received by the skin which can produce a severe skin reaction known as 'radiation burn'. Such damage is exacerbated by the radiation scatter produced when radiation strikes the skin surface and causes exposure of the area surrounding the treatment field and may increase the area of reaction.

Orthovoltage radiation with X-ray beams, generated between 150 and 500keV, is used when deeper penetration is needed; the majority of clinical applications rely on energies at between 200-300keV with the 90% dose within about 2cm of the skin surface (Williams and Thwaites, 1993). This enables treatment of deeper areas, such as breast tissue. However, the maximum dose is still received by the superficial tissues, such as the skin, so that erythema and desquamation may appear rapidly. Bone necrosis may also arise and is thought to be due to the fact that bone absorbs more orthovoltage radiation than does soft tissue (Hilderley, 1992). These effects may limit the total dose that can be given. The patient, or the radiation source, must be rotated so that the total dose is delivered through different entry points thus decreasing local toxicity.

Megavoltage therapy

Until the development of megavoltage equipment, skin toxicity was a common problem but, following its development, it became possible to generate radiation which does not produce its maximum dose at the skin surface but at a specific depth determined by the radiation energy generated by the unit employed.

Megavoltage equipment, operating between 2 and 40MeV, invokes a higher energy output and, therefore, deeper tissue penetration and, due to the greater dose-to-depth ratio, enables significant skin-sparing thus reducing skin toxicity and minimising subcutaneous

47

tissue destruction. The more homogeneous absorption of radiation also minimises the excessive absorption by bone that occurs in orthovoltage therapy thus reducing the incidence of bone necrosis (Hilderley, 1992). At the same time, the capacity for a higher output (radiation per minute) allows treatment of larger fields over shorter treatment periods and results in less radiation scatter. However, due to the higher energy and greater penetration, there is a risk of tissue damage (toxicity) at the exit site as well as the site of entry of the radiation beam(s).

The Cobalt-60 machine (1-4MeV), once the most commonly used megavoltage unit, can be used to treat tumours at most sites. Radioactive cobalt (^{60}Co) is a high energy radiation source which emits γ rays and is particularly useful in treating tumours of the head, neck, breast and metastatic lymph node involvement. However, because ^{60}Co is a radioactive isotope, it is undergoing constant decay. This necessitates monthly correction of the output to allow for the decay. The $t_{1/2}$ of 5.3 years means that the source must be changed every 5 years if lengthy treatment times are to be avoided.

Linear accelerators have become the treatment machines of choice in most radiotherapy units (Almond and Horton, 1993). They have marked advantages which include the speed at which treatment can be given and the ability to treat a sharply-defined treatment field thus exposing only the desired tissue volume to irradiation. These factors reduce the time that patients must lie in awkward positions and may also reduce the effects of radiation at the skin surface.

Supervoltage machines

Even more powerful linear accelerators, producing either X-ray or electron beams, can generate radiation at energies between 4-35MeV. Since the penetration of this radiation is great it is possible to treat tumours located several centimetres below the skin surface. In addition to the depth of penetration and its skin-sparing action, supervoltage therapy also reduces radiation scatter to adjacent tissues due to the high energy transfer. Its effect is to decrease both the incidence and severity of radiation sickness since this is related to the volume of body tissue receiving significant amounts of radiation.

Electrons, negatively charged particles, have a very small mass as a result of which they are easily deflected from their path by other electrons. This means that the depth to which they can penetrate a tissue is limited. As a result, electron beam therapy is primarily used to treat relatively superficial lesions, such as those of the skin or the chest wall; it is also useful in providing a 'booster' dose of radiation to a limited site following megadosage therapy (Hilderley, 1992).

High energy radiation

Two basic forms of radiation are used with therapeutic intent. These are: low linear energy transfer radiation (low LET), such as X-rays, γ rays and electrons, and high LET radiations such as neutron or proton beams, heavy ions (e.g. helium) and negative pi-mesons (Griffin, 1987). High LET radiations have advantages since they result in the deposition of large doses of radiation in small volumes of tissue while sparing adjacent normal tissues. They are also more effective against hypoxic cells which are usually relatively resistant to conventional therapy and result in decreased fluctuation in radio-sensitivity throughout the cell cycle (Griffin, 1987); there is also a reduction in the ability to repair sublethal cellular damage. In other words, they display greater biological effectiveness.

ADMINISTRATION OF TELETHERAPY

Radiation is directed from the source to the target area through an opening in the therapy machine (collimator). Lead blocks, attached to the collimator, are carefully positioned to 'block' the path of the radiation beam so that it affects only the defined target area. Alternatively, lead shielding may be applied directly to the body, again to protect normal tissues.

The pathway and penetration of the beam can be modified using filters or bolus bags (these are of a similar density to body tissue) (Williams and Thwaites, 1993). These techniques ensure that an accurate radiation dose is delivered to the defined target area and help to minimise radiation-induced side-effects in adjacent normal tissues.

To ensure continued accuracy and consistency of treatment the field is usually outlined with indelible ink, or small tattoos. Care must be taken by both the nursing staff and the patient to preserve these markings since maintaining the accuracy of the treatment field is critical if therapy is to be administered effectively and safely. Studies have shown that dose variations of only 5% can significantly affect survival (e.g. Lowry, 1974; Nias, 1990). This means that the patient must remain in exactly the same position during each period of treatment. When positioning is difficult a variety of techniques can be employed to maintain immobility for the required period. For example, individually made plaster casts or moulds can be used and tailored to meet individual requirements.

The choice of treatment appropriate to the patient's needs is, as has been shown, a product of three major factors: the tumour type, the stage of disease and the therapeutic objective.

Delivery of the radiation beams

External radiation is delivered in beams which may be directed in a number of different and/or intersecting planes and angles to ensure delivery of the appropriate dose to the tumour. A single radiation beam may be satisfactory in a limited number of cases but a midline tumour may be better treated through a pair of parallel opposed fields (Figure 4.2).

Figure 4.2   **Parallel opposed fields**

Radiation source

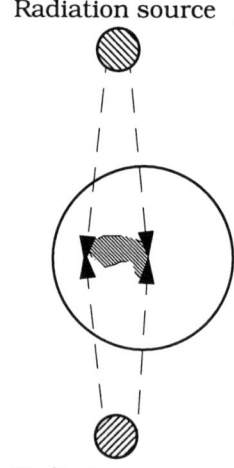

Radiation source

Alternatively rotation therapy may be employed when the machine usually rotates around the patient although the converse is also possible. However, there are times when, although rotation therapy is not appropriate, more than two approaches are required; in this case multiple field therapy is used (Figure 4.3).

Figure 4.3   **Multiple field therapy**

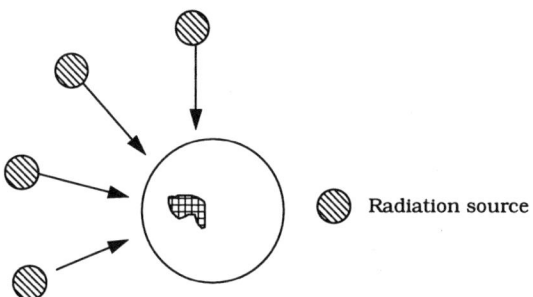

Radiation source

In cases where the radiation beams overlap, for example when two fields directed at right angles to each other are necessary, wedge filters are used to 'turn' the beam and eliminate 'hot spots' in over-lapping area(s). All radiation fields must be treated at each therapy session to ensure an even biological dose pattern.

BRACHYTHERAPY (Plesiotherapy) (See Chapter 13).
Brachytherapy is the term used to describe the administration of radiation via a radioactive source that is placed in, or in close proximity to, the tumour or tumour bed. This is achieved by either permanent or temporary implantation of a radioactive source in or near the tumour since, by placing the radiation source in, or immediately adjacent to, the volume of tissue to be treated the dose to other tissues can be minimised.

Although, in theory, brachytherapy may be used to treat tumours at any site, in practice its use is currently, limited to easily accessible sites either near the body surface or in/near a natural body cavity. Developments in intra-operative radiotherapy may lead to increasing use of this technique. Brachytherapy may be used as the sole method of treatment; it may also be combined with teletherapy or used either pre-or post-operatively.

Radioactive sources may be loaded into applicators specially made to fit into body cavities, inserted directly into tumours and if the source is a short-lived isotope, it may be left as a permanent implant. The most common radioactive sources used in brachytherapy are cobalt-60 (^{60}Co), caesium-137 (^{137}Cs), iridium-192 (^{192}Ir), tantalum-182 (^{182}Ta) and gold-198 (^{198}Au); radium-226 (^{226}Ra), Yttrium-90 (^{90}Y) and iodine-125 (^{125}I) are also used. The techniques used may be divided into three groups: interstitial implants, intracavity implants

51

Use of radiation to treat cancer

and mould or applicator treatment and are described as sealed sources of radiation.

Interstitial implants

Using this technique the radioactive source is implanted directly into the cancerous tissue and the tumour bed. A high radiation dosage is provided in or near the tumour which rapidly diminishes in the regions outside the tumour. There is, however, an intensely high, although localised, zone of irradiation immediately around each implant. In general, this is advantageous and, as a result, interstitial therapy is ideally suited for anatomical situations in which the tumour is well-localised in accessible tissues, such as the tongue or lip. However, implantation can be carried out at open surgery for inaccessible tumours such as those of the bladder or prostate.

The type of implant used is dependent on the thickness and size of the tumour. Small lesions, up to 0.5cm in diameter, can be treated by a single plane implant; larger tumours require two or more planes. Volume implants are used for tumours more than 2.5cm thick.

Caesium-137, ^{192}Ir, ^{182}Ta), ^{198}Au and ^{90}Y and are the isotopes most commonly used in interstitial therapy although some units also use ^{226}Ra. Implants may be in the form of needles, wires, seeds or grains. Needles, wires and ribbons are particularly useful in treating lesions of the head and neck. Needle heads have eyes through which threads are tied. These serve two purposes. Firstly they enable regular counting of the number of threads and, therefore, the number of needles present and, secondly, they are used for removing the needles. Tumour tissue necrosis around the needle means that traction on the threads will allow easy removal.

Seeds or grains are particularly useful for treatment of intra-abdominal or intrathoracic lesions when the seeds are introduced either through hollow needles or tubes or by means of a 'seed gun' which injects the sources directly into the tumour. Such sources are usually permanent so that radiation precautions may be necessary for some time after implantation dependent on the half life of the radioisotope concerned (see Ch 13).

Afterloading techniques, designed to reduce the exposure of staff to radiation, have been developed. Such techniques require insertion of empty source containers into the tissues or a body cavity; the radioactive sources can then be loaded later. The advantage of this approach is that care can be taken to ensure appropriate placement and radiographic studies used to confirm the position of the containers, without unnecessary exposure of those staff involved. The sources are inserted into the applicator when all the necessary checks have been made and the patient has returned to the ward. This is particularly important in relation to the relatively strong sources used for intracavity treatment (Easson and Pointon, 1985). Thus afterloading both ensures that implantation is accurate and that an even dose of radiation is delivered to the tumour and facilitates removal of the source on completion of treatment.

Two methods of afterloading are in use: automatic (remote) and manual techniques. Using automatic techniques, the sources are contained in a lead safe by the patient's bed on the ward; they can be loaded automatically into the applicator from outside the room (Aird and Williams, 1993). The catheters or containers are connected to a machine, such as the Selectron, which can rapidly insert the sources or withdraw them into a shielded container when required thus reducing the exposure of the staff. Use of this technique, however, requires complex and sophisticated equipment if it is not to lead to less accurate and inferior treatment.

Alternatively, manual techniques may be employed when the sources are mounted on long flexible handles which enable them to be pushed into position. The main disadvantage is that, although theatre staff will receive no radiation, the ward staff are still exposed to radiation during nursing and other procedures. However, application of the principles of shielding, time of exposure and distance from the source will reduce exposure of all those involved.

Despite its value afterloading is not essential since, when working with preloaded applicators, careful attention to working procedures and the use of appropriate handling and shielding can restrict the exposure of all the staff involved to levels below the acceptable occupational dose limits (see Ch 2) (Easson and Pointon, 1985). However, exposure can still range between 30% and 90% of the permissible dose (Easson and Pointon, 1985) and may fail to meet the requirements of the International Commission on Radiological Protection that states that exposure should not only be less than the permissible dose limit but also 'as low as reasonable achievable'.

Intracavity implants

Intracavity implants involve the placement of a radioactive source into a body cavity for the purpose of treating malignant disease in or around that cavity. This technique is most commonly used in the treatment of gynaecological cancers, such as those of the vagina, cervix and uterus. Applicators are inserted in surgery; the radioactive material may then be inserted at that time or by use of afterloading techniques.

A variety of techniques and equipment have been developed to provide the required dosage of radiation to the tissues around the radiation source (Shell and Carter, 1987). Most of those used in treating gynaecological malignancies are based on the 'Manchester method' described below.

The Manchester Method (Easson and Pointon, 1985): Using this approach the radioactive source is contained in two vaginal ovoids separated by a spacer; a central uterine tube is added when both the cervix and the body of the uterus are to be treated.

It is usual to administer 2 applications, of approximately 72 hours each, at 4 day intervals. This ensures that a constant radiation dose is delivered to the para-cervical region. The source used is usually caesium-137.

The Stockholm Technique: This method of treatment is fractionated so that it is usual for three treatments, of 22 hours each, to be spread over a period of 3-4 weeks. Again the radioisotope chosen is usually caesium-137 which is loaded into a uterine tube that fills the uterine cavity from the fundus to the external cervical os. Box-shaped applicators are inserted into the vagina against the external os. The dose delivered to the bladder and rectum is measured and, provided this is satisfactory, treatment continues.

Alternatively, the uterus may be packed using small capsules of radioactive material until the cavity is filled. Each capsule has a metal thread running from it and a numbered tag on the end of the thread. This enables easy removal of the capsules and permits checking of the number of capsules in situ. The capsules are left in position until a total dose of 60Gy is administered to the whole of the uterine wall. This method of treatment may be repeated once.

Mould/applicator treatments (surface therapy)

Such therapy is often classified as a type of brachytherapy because it involves close contact between the source and the malignant lesion (Hilderley, 1992). Any radioactive source may be used in this form of treatment being mounted onto a moulded base that is applied directly to the body surface. Moulds are individually made for each patient, the source being 'sandwiched' between two layers of a special plastic and then applied to the body surface. The aim is to deliver a stated dose to the skin surface at a fixed distance from the source; the advantage is that curved or irregular surfaces can be homo-geneously treated. Since the rays do not penetrate deeply into the tissues moulds are used only to treat thin, superficial tumours such as basal or squamous cell tumours of the skin, mouth, lip or cheek.

Treatment may be continuous or discontinuous. Moulds used for continuous treatment are designed to stay in place throughout the entire treatment period and are usually adhesive. A discontinuous mould is designed to be worn for a calculated time each day for the defined treatment period, usually 8 days although this is dependent of the strength of the source. This approach is, therefore, particularly suitable for use in older people and, since it may be used at home, those who would find daily treatment in the hospital difficult.

This was formerly an important area of sealed source therapy since the rapid fall-off in dose made it particularly appropriate for treatment of superficial tumours lying above sensitive normal tissues. However, its usefulness has diminished with the increasing availability of electron therapy units (Aird and Williams, 1993).

SYSTEMIC RADIATION (Unsealed source therapy)

Radioactive substances may be administered in liquid form by the intravenous or the oral route. They may be infused into or lymphatic system or instilled into a body cavity. Such therapy has been in use for over 50 years and, in certain cases, can deliver a larger internal dose of radiation to target tissues more effectively than external beam therapy (Flower and Chittenden, 1993). For example, instillation of yttrium-90 into the pleural or peritoneal cavity can significantly reduce the accumulation of a pleural effusion or recurrent ascites, particularly when used in conjunction with systemic drug therapy.

An alternative approach is to choose an element that can be concentrated by the body into one particular area. Good examples are iodine which is taken up by the thyroid gland or phosphorus which concentrates in the bone marrow.

Iodine-131 is the most commonly used unsealed source of radiation. It produces some γ rays and is, therefore, useful in producing a scan picture of the thyroid. However, most of its irradiation is emitted as β rays which has led to its major use in treating diseases of the thyroid as it will deliver a high dose of radiation to the gland. It is administered by mouth as a colourless and tasteless solution of sodium iodide and, like dietary iodide, it is taken up by the thyroid. Any iodine not taken up in this way is rapidly excreted in the urine so that the dose of radiation received by the rest of the body is negligible.

However, in some cases, the dose of a radionuclide that can be delivered to a tumour is limited by the maximum dose that can be tolerated by normal tissues. For example, in systemic therapy, the dose-limiting organ is often the bone marrow so that, when there is a known risk of bone marrow damage, a bone marrow harvest may be performed prior to therapy for subsequent regrafting should this prove necessary (Flower and Chittenden, 1993). A high uptake of particular radioisotopes by the liver could result in radiation hepatitis and/or chronic veno-occlusive disease. Further details are presented in Chapter 12.

REFERENCES

Almond PR, Horton JL, 1993, Planning and acceptance testing of megavoltage therapy installations. In: Williams JR, Thwaites DI (Editors), Radiotherapy Physics in Practice, Oxford Medical Publications, Oxford.

Dietz K, 1979, Radiation therapy: external radiation, Cancer Nursing, **2**, 233-244.

Easson EC, Pointon RCS, 1985, The Radiotherapy of Malignant Disease, Springer-Verlag, New York.

Flower MA, Chittender SJ, 1993, Unsealed source therapy. In: Williams JR, Thwaites DI, (Editors), Radiotherapy Physics in Practice, Oxford Medical Publications, Oxford, 1993.

Griffin TW, 1987, High linear energy transfer and heavy charged particles. In: Perez CA, Brady LW (Editors), Principles and Practice of Radiation Oncology, JB Lippincott Co, Philadelphia.

Hall D, 1995, New ideas on fractionation and accelerated radio-therapy, Nursing Times, **91**(12), 42-43.

Hilderley LJ, 1992, Radiotherapy. In: Groenwald SL, Frogge MH, Goodman M, Yarbro CH, (Editors), Treatment Modalities. Part III from Cancer Nursing: Principles and Practice (Second edition), Jones and Bartlett Publishers, Boston.

Klevenhagen SC, Thwaites DI, 1993, Kilovoltage X-rays. In: Williams

JR, Thwaites DI (Editors), Radiotherapy Physics in Practice, Oxford Medical Publications, Oxford.

Lowry S, 1974, Fundamentals of Radiation Therapy, English Universities Press, London.

Nias AHW, 1990, An Introduction to Radiobiology, John Wiley and Sons, Chichester.

Parker R, 1980, Principles of radiation oncology. In: Haskell C (Editor), Cancer Treatment, WB Saunders Co., Philadelphia.

Redpath AT, Williams JR, Thwaites DI, 1993, Treatment planning for external beam therapy. In: Williams JR, Thwaites DI (Editors), Radiotherapy Physics in Practice, Oxford Medical Publications, Oxford.

Saunders MI, Dische J, 1986, Radiotherapy employing three fractions each day over a continuous period of 12 days, British Journal of Radiology, **59**, 523-525.

Shell J, Carter J, 1987, The gynecological implant patient, Seminars in Oncology Nursing, **3**(1), 54-68.

van Eys J, 1987, Living beyond cure: transcendng survival, American Journal of Pediatric Haematology and Oncology, **9**, 114-118.

Williams JR, Thwaites DI, Introduction. In: Williams JR, Thwaites DI, (Editors), Radiotherapy Physics in Practice, Oxford Medical Publications, Oxford, 1993.

CHAPTER 5   THE PATIENT AS AN INDIVIDUAL

An individual approach to the care of patients undergoing radio-therapy is essential since they must be recognised as 'individuals experiencing a special and severe form of stress' (Schneider, 1978) which is related both to the disease itself and the treatment they are to receive. No aspect of the patient's life remains unaffected by the disease. Indeed, it is widely acknowledged that cancer is 'one of the most feared and stressful of all diseases' (Jalowiec and Dudas 1991). As a result, the development of cancer poses a severe threat not only to the physical welfare of patients but also to their psychological condition. Since nurses have the most consistent and continuing relationship with the patient they are in the ideal position to help him to come to terms with his difficulties. A thorough nursing assess-ment, designed to provide information about both actual and potential problems, is essential and will help them to identify appropriate interventions.

In carrying out such an assessment it must be recognised that each cancer patient is unique having his own personality traits and his own personal circumstances (McGee, 1991). This means that the meaning of the disease, and the person's interpretation of it, is also unique. An individual assessment implies a willingness to listen to the patient and his family to identify their needs, concerns and anxieties about the disease and its treatment. It will also enable these factors to be placed in the context of the patient's understanding of his disease. Thus, a truly individual approach focuses on the individual well-being and helps to develop an understanding of the patient and to enhance his dignity and self-esteem; it will also help to increase his confidence and trust in the health care team.

The cancer patient is required to make numerous decisions many of which relate either to treatment options or to adaptation to the various changes in lifestyle which, almost inevitably, follow the diagnosis of cancer and/or the start of treatment. Daily treatment, combined with the stress of disease, disrupts the normal pattern of activity and can cause profound and distressing anxiety and concern.

Responses to the diagnosis of cancer are often compounded by reactions to its treatment; it must, therefore, be recognised that patients facing radiotherapy are often very vulnerable, particularly when this commences within a short time of diagnosis. Following diagnosis many patients suffer overwhelming feelings of loss of control which may, in turn, lead to feelings of both helplessness and hopelessness and a belief that they have no influence over what is happening to them. Alternatively, irradiation may be the last in a long line of debilitating treatments when the prevailing feelings may be despair and anger. Many have a profound fear of radiation which is based, in part, on old wives' tales and also on its association with nuclear technology. For others, it may confirm the diagnosis of cancer or provide a forceful reminder that their disease is malignant (Bond, 1982) or be viewed as a 'last resort'.

As a method of treatment, radiation cannot be seen or felt yet it causes various degrees of discomfort which can be difficult for the patient to understand. It is delivered by machines which are large, unfamiliar and noisy and the patient must lie in an uncomfortable position on a hard bed whilst he is 'bombarded' with irradiation. As a result, radiotherapy has been found to be a considerable source of emotional distress, anxiety and depression (e.g. Peck and Boland, 1977; Forester et al, 1978; Silberfarb et al, 1980).

Understanding can help the patient to maintain an element of control so that many will seek information in an attempt to reduce the uncertainty surrounding both the diagnosis and the treatment. Cassileth et al (1980), however, suggested that, although patients frequently sought information, this was not always forthcoming. They also found that most patients wanted the maximum amount of information. Those seeking detailed information were predominantly younger, better educated and more recently diagnosed than those who avoided information and who wanted others to make decisions for them.

However, although most patients want information, and find this beneficial, some researchers believe that giving information when this is not wanted may disrupt denial mechanisms leading to a loss of hope and even depression (e.g. Bloom et al, 1978; Kellerman et al, 1980). This has been supported by Gotay (1984) and Hopkins (1986) who found that those with advanced disease were likely to seek less information than those with more limited disease attributing this to the self-protective use of denial and avoidance mechanisms. This suggests that the provision of information is not always a desirable aim of care and stresses the need to treat each patient as an individual and assess his need or desire for information.

The kind of information wanted by patients has also been

investigated (e.g. Derdiarian 1986, 1987; Cassileth et al 1980) showing that the majority of those wanting information wanted this to be related to the disease itself as well as that related to the side-effects of treatment(s), treatment outcomes and the potential for cure. However, although many patients would welcome the opportunity to discuss their situation more fully, many felt it was not appropriate to do so with the staff with whom they most commonly come into contact (i.e. the medical, nursing and technical staff) often believing that the staff are 'too busy' to 'waste time' talking to them (e.g. Holmes and Dickerson 1987).

This highlights the challenge to be faced in helping patients to reach understanding of their disease and its treatment and, perhaps, goes some way towards explaining the burgeoning interest in self-help groups and complementary approaches to cancer treatment. It must, however, be recognised that not all radiotherapy out-patient departments enjoy the benefits of a regular nursing staff so that much of the supportive care, particularly for outpatients, falls to the radiographers whose time is limited.

The most effective means of meeting those needs is through carefully planned patient education which takes individual needs into account. It is probable that, as suggested by Muntz and Zur (1978) 'in no other illness is the need for continued and supportive education so necessary'. The educative process with regard to radio-therapy must include explanation of the treatment process itself, of the machines to be employed and of the need for immobilisation which, although uncomfortable, usually lasts only a few minutes. An opportunity should also be created to enable the patient to express his fears and anxieties about his disease and treatment which will, in turn, create the opportunity for nursing interventions with regard to the provision of appropriate information and psychological and/or emotional support. A tour of the treatment area prior to the start of treatment may prove valuable. These actions can significantly increase patient understanding, enhance compliance and improve the quality of the patient's life.

Despite the many precautions which are taken some degree of damage to normal tissues is inevitable although this occurs only when these are included in the treatment field. Knowledge of the tolerance of normal tissues will help carers to anticipate the onset and severity of likely side-effects and to prepare the patient for their occurrence. Such effects often make the patient feel worse physically than they did before treatment started and side-effects are commonly misinterpreted as a progression of their disease.

As side-effects rarely arise during the first two weeks of treatment a systematic teaching plan can help to prepare the patient and to teach him suitable and simple self-care measures. Involving the patient in his treatment can help to decrease unnecessary morbidity and demonstrates the important role they can play in their own care and treatment. Cassileth et al (1980) have shown that the most hopeful patients are those who are actively involved in their care. The importance of patient participation cannot be stressed highly enough since this helps them to feel more in control; this forms the basis of many of the 'alternative' approaches to cancer care and, perhaps, accounts for some of the increasing interest in these approaches.

Since Jacobs et al (1983) have shown that appropriate education decreases anxiety and reduces the incidence of treatment-related problems, depression and disruption of the life-style, education should be regarded as a vital component of total patient care. If health care professionals are to carry this out effectively they must develop their own level of understanding so that simple but accurate explanations can be given. Thus they must, themselves, be aware of the experiences to which the patient will be exposed. Some of these are considered briefly below.

THE TREATMENT PROCESS

Due to the radiation hazards which may be posed to the staff, and to the environment, it is usual for the radiotherapy department to be in a remote part of the hospital complex; the walls are constructed of thick concrete. Its remote position and unusual construction may confirm the patient's fears of radiation. It is, therefore, important that explanations include not only the expected therapeutic outcome but also the reason for such protective measures.

The way in which the therapeutic plan will be constructed must be described, together with the fact that, during treatment planning he must lie absolutely still, sometimes in uncomfortable positions. The importance of skin markings must be stressed. Skin markings can serve as a constant reminder of the presence of malignancy and so can be a marked source of distress particularly when the treatment field includes an area of the body which is constantly exposed; permanent tattoos may cause continued distress long after treatment has been completed.

The patient as an individual

Many patients are very anxious about the process associated with their treatment; this may be exacerbated by the fact that they are to be left alone during the treatment period. Use of an intercom can do much to reassure the patient as can assurances that he will be observed throughout his treatment either by means of a television monitor or through a leaded glass (shielded) window. They must be warned that first treatment will take longer than subsequent treatments since the therapeutic plan will be checked to ensure that the entire tumour is included in the treatment field. Although the treatment session is short, the treatment table is hard and flat and lying immobile may cause pain or discomfort; where necessary analgesics should be given an hour beforehand to ensure that the patient is comfortable and as relaxed as possible during his therapy.

Wherever possible, the patient's treatment will be given at the same time(s) on each of the treatment days. Before the course of treatment commences the patient will be informed how many therapy sessions are necessary; the importance of receiving the prescribed dose must be stressed. Where disruption of the schedule is unavoidable adjustments are made to the original treatment plan to compensate for omitted treatments. These may include an increased dose over the remaining treatments or an extension of the original course of treatment. Changes may also be made as treatment progresses as a result of monitoring the tumour. The reasons underlying such changes must be explained to the patient.

ANXIETY AND LEARNING

Staff must be aware of the patient's anxiety level as this may limit both retention and understanding and affect the amount of information that can be given. This will also be affected by the patient's previous knowledge, understanding and beliefs about both cancer and radiation. These, combined with fear and anxiety, may lead to a failure to ask questions and seek clarification about what is to happen to them; this, in itself, may be indicative of stress. The initial assessment will have identified some of the patient's beliefs so that these can be taken into account when planning an appropriate teaching programme.

Other factors to be taken into account include the ability of the health care professional to teach what the patient needs to know and the recognition of that need by the patient. It must be remembered that an individual will only learn what he needs or wants to know so that learning/teaching goals must be set with the patient. At the same time, his priorities may change as treatment progresses so that continued reassessment and evaluation of the teaching plan is essential. The patient's motivation provides the key to his willingness to learn so that the first task is to motivate him whilst, at the same time, establishing his needs, wants and worries as these are central to the learning process. Teaching will not be successful unless it involves the patient.

This approach permits the patient to play an active role in his learning and will help to build trust between the carer and the patient and help him to maintain his dignity and self-esteem. Such a relationship will encourage the patient to ask questions and seek the information that he requires. It should also be remembered that repetition strengthens learning; positive feedback and reinforcement are, therefore, essential.

Thus, if our teaching is to be successful, we must first identify what is needed and help the patient to interpret the facts and identify possible courses of action based on these. The success of teaching can be evaluated by the role the patient is able to play in his care and the quality of his life when he returns to his usual environment. It is also indicative of the quality of care he receives.

Basic steps

Once the goals of teaching/learning have been established the basic steps outlined below will simplify the teaching process.

- Tell the patient what information is to be covered during each teaching session.
- Organise the information into related categories; cover the most important information first.
- Keep the teaching sessions short.
- Keep the information simple, use short words and sentences which are easily understood. Avoid the use of 'jargon'.
- Summarise and review the material covered.

However, not all teaching need be formalised since the patient may ask direct questions which must be answered. Nurses, in particular, have many opportunities to talk to patients and can use these to exchange information. Informal teaching of this type has a valuable role to play and can signify motivation and interest on behalf of the patient. It also helps to demonstrate the nurse's interest in the patient as an individual.

The patient as an individual

The last, and most important, step is evaluation which is, all too often, forgotten. It cannot be assumed that information given is retained and understood; teaching does not, in itself, equate with learning. As a result, teaching must be evaluated to ensure that the patient understands the information and can relate it, or apply it, to his own situation.

Evaluation allows care to be dynamic and, as such, subject to continued change and reassessment. Each patient requires an individual approach as both the beneficial and the side-effects of radiation must be assessed and appropriate interventions planned and implemented. These are discussed in detail in subsequent chapters. Concurrent evaluation will be carried out by the physician and the radiotherapists and appropriate adjustments made to the treatment plan.

Following radiotherapeutic treatment of malignant disease it is important that consistent, long term follow-up is carried out. This enables monitoring of both individual progress and the incidence of late side-effects of radiation since some of these may not develop for some 5-10 years or longer after cessation of treatment (see Ch 6). The patient should be encouraged to attend as instructed and assured that follow-up care is planned not because a recurrence of the disease is expected (although this may be the case in palliative treatment) but simply to monitor his progress. However, if the disease should return, regular examination should enable early detection and an improved chance of control.

NEEDS OF NURSES INVOLVED CARING FOR RADIOTHERAPY PATIENTS

Since nurses are required to help patients to express their problems and fears, and to develop an environment conducive to communication and support, it is essential that they are, themselves, provided with the appropriate skills and training and also have access to appropriate methods of support. Without effective inter-personal skills nurses may feel uncomfortable in communicating with patients and may experience marked difficulties in meeting patient needs with regard to information and emotional support.

Nurses, like any other individuals, require help in sharing their feelings and their reactions to patients which will, in turn, help their approach to problem solving both on a personal level and with regard to the patients in their care.

However, communication among staff can be as difficult as that between staff and patients and nurses have been shown to work in relative emotional isolation such that Vachon et al (1978) have shown that stress in nurses can be considerably higher than that of patients beginning treatment for breast cancer and only slightly lower than that of new widows. Yet, to disclose such feelings to peers would mean admitting to what may be thought to be an 'unprofessional attitude' so that there may be an understandable reluctance to share responses and to identify not only the need for help in resolving difficulties on an individual basis but also a failure to appreciate that there may be common difficulties to be faced and overcome (Bond, 1982). This is important not only in relation to the difficulties faced by staff but also to patients since Cassee (1975) has shown that open socio-emotional communication between staff and patient is less likely to occur when there is an absence of staff communication on an emotional level.

Thus a support network for staff can only be beneficial to patient care. Regular, multidisciplinary staff meetings can be helpful in providing a mutually supportive environment, particularly when this is facilitated by a psychologist who can both help the staff to cope with their own problems as well as those of the patients in their care.

REFERENCES

Bloom JR, Ross RD, Burnell G, 1978, The effect of social support on patient adjustment after breast surgery, Patient Counselling and Health Education, **2**, 50-59.

Bond S, 1982, Communication in cancer nursing. In: Cahoon MC, Cancer Nursing, Recent Advances in Nursing 3, Churchill Livingstone, Edinburgh.

Cassee E, 1975, Therapeutic behaviour, hospital culture and communication. In: Cox C, Mead A (Editors), A Sociology of Medical Practice, Collier MacMillan, London.

Cassileth B, Zupkis R, Sutton-Smith K, 1980, Informed consent - why are its goals imperfectly realised? New England Journal of Medicine, **302**, 896-900.

Derdiarian AK, 1986, Informational needs of recently diagnosed cancer patients, Nursing Research, **35**, 276-281.

Derdiarian AK, 1987, Informational needs of recently diagnosed cancer patients, Part II, Method and description, Cancer Nursing, **10**, 156-163.

Forester B M, Kornfeld DS, Fleiss J, 1978, Psychiatric effects of radiotherapy, American Journal of Psychiatry, **135**, 900 - 963.

Gotay CC, 1984, The experience of cancer during early and advanced stages: the views of patients and their mates, Social Science and Medicine, **18**, 605-613.

Holmes S, Dickerson JWT, 1987, The quality of life: design and evaluation of a self-assessment instrument for use with cancer patients, International Journal of Nursing Studies, **24**, 15-24.

Hopkins MB, 1986, Information-seeking and adaptational outcomes in women receiving chemotherapy for breast cancer, Cancer Nursing, **9**, 256-262.

Jacobs C, Ross R, Walker L, Stockdale F, 1983, Behaviour of cancer patients: a randomised study of the effects of education and peer support groups, American Journal of Clinical Oncology (June) 347-350.

Jalowiec A, Dudas S, 1991, Alterations in patient coping. In Baird SB, McCorkle R, Grant M, (Editors), Cancer Nursing: A Comprehensive Textbook, WB Saunders Co., London.

Kellerman J, Riglee D, Siegel SE, Katz ER, 1980, Disease related communication and depression in pediatric patients, Journal of Pediatric Psychology, **2**, 52-53.

McGee RF, 1992, Overview of psychosocial dimensions, In: Groenwald SL, Frogge MH, Goodman M, Yarbro CH, (Editors) Part IV from Cancer Nursing. Principles and Practice, (Second edition), Jones and Bartlett Publishers, Boston.

Muntz ML, Zur BH, 1978, The role of the nurse in patient education. In: Kellogg CJ, Sullivan P (Editors), Current Perspectives in Oncolgic Nursing (Volume 2), CV Mosby, St Louis.

Peck A, Boland J, 1977, Emotional reactions to radiation treatment, Cancer, **40**, 180-184.

Schneider L, 1978 Identification of human concerns by cancer patients. In: Kellogg CJ, Sullivan BP (Editors), Current Perspectives in Oncolgic Nursing (Volume 2), C V Mosby, St Louis.

Silberfarb PM, Maurer LH, Crouhamel CS, 1980, Psychosocial aspects of neoplastic disease. 1. Functional status of breast cancer patients during different treatment regimens, American Journal of Psychiatry, **135**, 960 - 965

Vachon MLS, Lyall WAL, Freeman SJJ, 1978, Measurement and management of stress in health professionals working with advanced cancer patients, Death Education, **1**, 365-275.

CHAPTER 6   RADIATION-INDUCED SIDE-EFFECTS

Since the effects of radiation are not restricted only to malignant cell populations both normal and cancer cells may be affected although toxicity will affect only those cells included in the treatment field. However, most treatment fields encompass at least some normal tissue in order to allow an adequate safety margin and ensure that all malignant cells are included. When effects are exerted on normal cells, the signs and symptoms produced are described as the side-effects of radiotherapy. Generalised effects may also occur including fatigue, lethargy, nausea and vomiting; 'radiation sickness' or 'radiation syndrome' may also arise (p76).

Side-effects may occur days, months or even years after treatment depending on the tissues/organs irradiated and the treatment regime involved. The nature and severity of side-effects may be influenced by a variety of factors including:

- Amount of normal tissue included in the treatment field
- Tissues/organs included in the treatment field
- Radiosensitivity of tissues/organs involved
- Total dose of radiation administered
- Fractionation of the total dose
- Energy level of radiation employed
- Previous/concurrent chemotherapy or surgery
- Individual susceptibility dependent on age and general health.

This means that, although certain side-effects are to be expected, there is considerable individual variation in both their onset and their degree so that, for some patients, the effects may be hardly noticeable whereas, in others they may be severe.

Acute side-effects are those occurring during, or shortly after, treatment due to the immediate responses to radiation and are primarily related to the total dose employed and the degree of fractionation.

Acute reactions develop as a result of the effects of radiation on cell renewal (replication) and are, therefore, often increased in areas of rapid cellular turnover (e.g. skin, bone marrow and gastrointestinal tract). Such effects may not be severe but may, nevertheless, be difficult for patients to cope with; on occasion they may be so severe that the daily dose of radiation must be reduced or treatment interrupted to allow recovery to occur. Care is focused on minimising their severity and helping patients to come to terms with them whilst reinforcing the fact that symptoms do not, of necessity, indicate disease progression. Most are self-limiting and subside once treatment ceases and cell proliferation returns to normal.

Subacute side-effects occur weeks or months after treatment as a result of which they may be difficult to differentiate from disease progression.

The total therapeutic dose of radiation and the time:dose relationship largely determine the incidence of intermediate side-effects particularly in tissues with a slow rate of cell turnover (e.g. endothelial tissues) when damage may not occur until some months after treatment. The patient may require considerable support and reassurance at this time. Anticipation and prompt recognition of such effects can allow rapid treatment and prevent serious complications.

Late/chronic responses may arise 1-5 years (or longer) after exposure. They are related to the total therapeutic dose received by tissues which, although slowly dividing, are particularly radio-sensitive. Although they may be related to previous acute or subacute side-effects they may also appear to be unrelated to either the occurrence or severity of acute reactions. Effects include tissue necrosis, fistulae and dense fibrosis which, unlike acute reactions, are not always amenable to treatment. They may be irreversible causing chronic symptoms. The care provided must be symptomatic and based on the degree of functional impairment. Carcinogenesis is another potential complication that may not be seen for many years after exposure (see p76-77).

SYMPTOM MANAGEMENT

The management of radiation-induced side-effects primarily falls to nurses. Since radiation is a localised treatment, the effects are also localised and can, to some extent at least, be predicted. This means that patients can often be prepared for their occurrence and taught appropriate self-care measures designed to minimise their impact.

This does not mean that there are no generalised (or systemic) effects. Again, the patient can benefit from being told what effects may arise as a result of his therapy. This may help to enable him to differentiate between radiation-induced effects and those which may indicate further progression of his disease.

Skin reactions

Despite the use of 'skin-sparing' techniques (supervoltage and mega-voltage machines), and regardless of the site receiving radiation, some degree of skin reaction is likely in patients undergoing radiotherapy since radiation must pass through the skin before reaching the target area. Depending on the type and energy of the radiation employed, the skin at the exit site may also be affected. Factors that increase the risk of skin reactions are shown in Table 6.1.

Table 6.1   Factors which increase the risk of skin reactions

The total dose of radiation given
The fractionation regime
The volume of the treatment field
The use of radiosensitising drugs such as adriamycin
The area/volume treated

As the epithelium comprises rapidly dividing cells some will be damaged or destroyed as radiation enters and leaves the treatment field. Some areas of the skin are particularly vulnerable to radiation such as those where two skin surfaces are in contact (e.g. face, perineum) or where skin integrity has been disrupted (e.g. surgical wounds). Movement and tight, chafing clothing may exacerbate the irritation and moisture and warmth may make this particularly vulnerable to infection.

Skin reactions vary from very mild erythema to moist desquamation; some patients display no skin changes. They are, however, generally progressive increasing in intensity throughout the course of treatment. Initially, a sensation of warmth may be felt in the treated area but the first real indication of a reaction is erythema; this is not usually seen until about the third week of treatment. This is similar to that seen following exposure to sunlight and the colour may vary from a mild reddening to marked inflammation due to capillary dilation; slight oedema may also be present. Such reactions may progress to give a tanned appearance that, unlike that following exposure to the sun, may be permanent. In some cases, erythema is the only manifestation of skin damage while, in others, this may progress to dry or moist desquamation. Such reactions may take some time to resolve and are unlikely to heal while radiotherapy continues.

Radiation-induced side-effects

When dry desquamation occurs the skin becomes very dry, due to destruction of the sebaceous and sweat glands, and there may be a loss of hair (epilation). The patient complains of itching, flaking and cracking of the skin which, although uncomfortable, does not usually necessitate discontinuation of treatment. Such reactions may be seen within 2-4 weeks of the start of treatment depending largely on the time:dose relationship and the total dose of radiation received.

This is, occasionally, followed by inflammation, oedema and moist desquamation which is characterised by the formation of blisters, exudative ulceration and/or loss of the epidermis, effects which leave a raw surface and resemble those following second degree burns. However, the skin-sparing effects of modern approaches to therapy mean that such reactions can largely be predicted. For example, those receiving electron beam therapy in the range of 5500-6000cGy are likely to experience severe skin reactions; hyperfractionation may also increase the risk of significant skin damage following treatment.

Such damage is acutely painful and therapy is discontinued to allow time for the skin to recover. Continuation of treatment at this time would result in severe ulceration and damage to the underlying structures. Even when treatment is discontinued, and the skin appears to have regained its normal appearance, permanent damage may result and be manifested by late changes, such as atrophy and fibrosis, telangiectasia and vascular impairment; the skin may take on a leathery appearance. On occasions, the late changes may progress to carcinogenesis.

Care of the patient experiencing a skin reaction

Delivery of care can be considered under 3 broad categories: before, during and after therapy. To be successful it is dependent on assessment and continued evaluation of the prescribed care and on successful patient education. Involving the patient in his care is essential for all those undergoing radiotherapy since, as has been shown, any patient may experience a skin reaction; his behaviours and actions may be of critical importance in the prevention of complications. Care is directed towards maintaining the integrity of the skin, preventing augmentation of radiation-induced effects and reducing irritation.

Before treatment commences the patient should be taught the fundamentals of skin care which are designed to maintain skin integrity whilst preventing irritation or stress to the skin surface.

Because moisture will enhance skin reactions the area should be kept clean and dry and the importance of preserving the treatment markings must be stressed; no attempt to replace skin markings should be made since the precise delineation of the treatment field is vital in determining the success or failure of therapy.

The area may be washed gently using tepid water and, although it is often suggested that soap should be avoided, there is some evidence to suggest that its use will have no detrimental effect (Campbell and Illingworth, 1992); a soft cloth and a gentle, patting motion are advised. The area should be patted dry using a soft towel and a baby dusting powder may be applied as this is soothing to irritated skin. Care must be taken to ensure such powder does not contain a metal base (such as zinc) as this may augment the effects of irradiation and potentiate any skin reaction. Similarly, perfumed creams/lotions should be avoided.

During treatment. Although exposure to the sun should be discouraged the affected area should, wherever possible, be exposed to the air. Extremes of temperature should be avoided (e.g. hot water bottles, heat pads or ice packs) even when this appears to be soothing. Clothing should be loose and non-constricting and harsh fabrics should not be worn; 100% cotton is ideal.

Cosmetics and lotions should not be used although a steroid cream, such as hydrocortisone 1%, may be prescribed when irritation is present and wheat germ oil or pure lanolin may be soothing and prevent skin breakdown. Such actions are necessary throughout the period of treatment and until any skin reaction has disappeared after its completion. However, although hydrocortisone may be useful in reducing inflammation and irritation it has been suggested that this may result in further thinning of the skin and an increased susceptibility to injury (Thomas, 1990). It is, nonetheless, useful when irritation is severe.

If moist desquamation occurs active care is required to reduce the risk of infection which is increased by the blistering and ulceration. A thin layer of hydrocortisone ointment may be applied and covered with a non-stick dressing or, alternatively, the site may be cleansed with half strength hydrogen peroxide and normal saline. The affected area must also be kept dry and may be covered with a non-constrictive, non-adhesive dressing although exposure to the air will be beneficial whenever this is possible. Since the inflammatory response may be masked by the erythema and oedema, induced by radiation, careful monitoring of the signs and symptoms of infection is essential and swabs should be sent for bacteriological examination whenever this is suspected. Systemic or topical anti-biotics will be prescribed if, and when, necessary.

After treatment. Wet/moist desquamation may persist, particularly in folds of skin, so that dry, non-adherent dressings may be required for some time after treatment. Alternatively, this may leave a scab which will adhere to the treated area; if this is removed it will simply renew itself and prolong the period required for healing to take place.

Erythema may persist taking some weeks to subside and, as a result, this may remain irritating and susceptible to friction. This means that the patient should continue to wear loose clothing so that damage is minimised.

The late changes induced by radiation may require further medical intervention and care to maximise function and preserve appearance. The skin included in the treatment field will always be both thinner and dryer than the rest of the skin and may also remain tanned. If this is in an exposed area it may prove difficult for the patient to accept. In addition, this sensitive skin may need continuing protection for example, by using an electric razor and minimising exposure to the sun. Each patient must determine his personal tolerance to the sun, or other irritating factors, and act accordingly. Damage to the vasculo-connective tissue may mean that this is incapable of effective repair and so may remain more vulnerable to infection and/or trauma.

RECALL PHENOMENON

Although this is not a true radiation reaction it is sufficiently common to warrant consideration here. Administration of certain chemotherapeutic agents, such as actinomycin-D and adriamycin, can reactivate or recall radiation skin reactions. Typically this will mimic the patterns of earlier skin reactions.

Patients undergoing such therapy must be carefully monitored for such a response. The care required is as previously described. Treatment is symptomatic. When necessary the drug dosage may be modified or the chemotherapeutic agent changed.

ANOREXIA

A decreased appetite is a common problem affecting many patients with cancer. Although its aetiology is not fully understood it is clear that it is a complex process involving many physiological and psychological factors that may be exacerbated by both the therapeutic and side-effects of radiotherapy (Table 6.2). As a result many patients undergoing such treatment will develop anorexia which, in turn, can have a significant impact on both the physiological and their psychological condition. Anorexia can also contribute to a marked decline in nutritional status so that aggressive nutritional support may be required, particularly since it is known that patients who are well nourished are better able to tolerate radiotherapy and experience fewer side-effects (see Ch 14).

Table 6.2 **Factors contributing to anorexia in radiotherapy patients**

Fatigue
Changes in taste sensation
Xerostomia
Mucositis/stomatitis
Oesophagitis
Nausea and vomiting
Diarrhoea or constipation
Emotional/psychological responses to disease or treatment
Changes in life-style
Factors resulting from the disease
Changes in taste sensation
Dysphagia
? Toxic products released by tumour cells
Metabolic disturbances

This means that attempts to persuade the patient to eat must be aggressive and persevering but compassionate. It must be recognised that the degree and extent of anorexia are subject to considerable individual variation and are also variable within the same individual at different times. Interventions which work initially may not work for that patient when attempted for the second or third time (Schnipper, 1985). Both the patient and his family may need considerable reassurance and support and must be assured that the loss of appetite and feelings of fullness (early satiety), which may follow just a few mouthfuls, are largely outside the patient's control.

The provision of food can be an important means of demonstrating

73

care and affection for loved ones so that its rejection can be regarded as hurtful and taken to signify rejection of the person rather than just the food. This can set up feelings of guilt at not eating and can lead to unnecessary pressures and tensions between the patient and his family. Appropriate family and patient teaching and counselling, and the setting of realistic goals, can both help to overcome such effects. Suitable interventions include:

- In view of the early satiety encourage frequent snacks every 2-3 hours
- Encourage the use of high protein, high energy foods which 'make every mouthful count' (i.e. use nutrient dense foods)
- Ensure that pain is well controlled and anticipate the need for analgesia so that the patient is not distracted from eating by the presence of pain
- Ensure nausea is well-controlled. Antiemetic therapy half an hour before meals may encourage food consumption
- Reduce unpleasant environmental stimuli to a minimum (e.g. bedpans or commodes and other unpleasant smells and sights. At home reduce cooking smells)
- Use wine, sherry or other alcoholic drinks as appetite stimulants
- Take note of taste changes and overcome these where possible (see Ch 7)
- Be flexible and enable the patient to eat when he is hungry. Many patients undergoing radiotherapy feel hungry at breakfast time prior to treatment. Ensure that they eat well at this time.

Although anorexia is a complex and disturbing symptom for both and the patient and his family there is considerable potential for minimising its effects (Schnipper, 1985). The nutritional care of the patient undergoing radiotherapy is discussed in Chapter 14.

FATIGUE

Although many patients are able to continue to work and enjoy their usual activities during the course of their treatment, others will experience varying degrees of fatigue and malaise during radiotherapy and for some time after its completion. Indeed, fatigue has been reported to be the most severe effect of radiotherapy, particularly during the last week of treatment (e.g. Andersen and Tewfik, 1985).

74

Affected patients will feel tired and weak and unable to accomplish much (Kobashi-Schoot et al, 1985) so that this will interfere with their interest and willingness to participate in 'normal' events. Such patients may require considerable reassurance that this is a normal reaction to radiotherapy and does not indicate a worsening of their condition.

Fatigue is usually experienced during the first week of treatment persisting until 2-4 weeks after its completion and is thought to arise for two main reasons; firstly, energy demand is increased both by the processes of malignancy itself and as a result of the increase in anabolism required to repair normal cells included in the treatment field. Secondly, as treatment proceeds the rate of cellular destruction is increased; this is associated with the release of waste products/cellular debris into the circulation.

Care is directed towards helping the patient to maintain an optimum level of activity consistent with his disease status. Additional rest and a reduction in the level of activity undertaken may, however, be required. This is achieved by a combination of direct intervention and patient education and priorities should be established which will determine the most appropriate ways in which the patient's energy will be expended. Before this can be achieved the patient must be carefully assessed to identify the factors contributing to his fatigue and the resultant changes in his lifestyle.

Interventions for patients suffering from fatigue

The goal of care is to help the patient to maintain the highest possible quality of life, To achieve this it is important that he is prepared for the possibility of the occurrence of fatigue since this may influence his perception of it. It is also important to develop understanding of the meaning of this symptom to the patient as this may affect his willingness or ability to take action to overcome its effects on particular areas of his life. For example, an individual who regards his work as important, and derives satisfaction from it but places a lower emphasis on his social or recreational activities, may find it more acceptable to suspend his participation in social activities than to take time away from work (Nail, 1992).

The patient should be taught to take measures that will help to conserve his energy so that he can continue with at least some of his normal work and/or social and recreational activities if this is what he wants to do. He should, for example, be taught to rest when tired and, particularly, following treatment; this is not always easy to achieve if he must travel a long way to the hospital for treatment. Periods of rest can be increased by, for example, going to bed early at night or, where possible, staying in bed later in the morning. Whereever possible, the patient should be encouraged to maintain his usual activities but, at the same time, he should be advised to pace himself to take account of his need for additional rest. Maintenance of a normal food intake, and optimal nutritional status, will help to boost his energy supply and help to reduce fatigue.

For those treated on an outpatient basis one of the most tiring factors is the daily attendance at the treatment centre since hospital transport can be slow and time consuming and, as such, extremely tiring (Sutcliffe and Holmes, 1991) Alternative means of transport should be explored to ensure that the patient has access to the easiest and most appropriate method of transport.

RADIATION SICKNESS (SYNDROME)

Radiotherapy can cause generalised symptoms that are not specifically related to the area being treated; these include fatigue, malaise, headache, nausea, vomiting and anorexia. It has been suggested that they result from absorption of tumour breakdown products (Bushke and Parker, 1972) although this has not been confirmed.

The severity of symptoms appears to be related to the volume of tissue included in the treatment field and the daily dose delivered; they must be carefully assessed since they may indicate the patient's radiation tolerance level. Adjustment of the treatment schedule, to include rest periods, combined with antiemetic and analgesic therapy, may help to alleviate the impact of the symptoms.

LATE EFFECTS OF RADIATION

Radiation may also result in late changes which occur some years after exposure; a latent period of 8-10 years (or even longer may be seen. Such changes represent the clinical manifestations of progressive degenerative processes induced by radiation (Nias, 1990) and largely depend on the number of parenchymal cells killed as well as the extent of ischaemia and fibrosis induced by radiation (Table 6.3). These are discussed further in later chapters.

Table 6.3 **Pathogenesis of early and late radiation effects**
(Nias, 1988)

Cell/tissue damaged	Damage	Effect
Early		
Differentiated cells	Cell depletion	Hypoplasia
Vascular endothelium	Increased permeability	Oedema
Late		
Differentiated cells	Cell depletion	Atrophy
Vascular endothelium	Increased permeability	Oedema
	Endarteritis	Fibrosis, ischaemia

There is also a great deal of concern about the carcinogenic effects of ionising radiation. The leukaemias are the most important neoplastic disease induced in this way (Nias, 1990). However, evidence also implicates radiation in the causation of some sarcomas, thyroid carcinoma and lung cancer (Hilderley, 1992).

Exposure to ionising radiations certainly increases the natural rate of malignant transformations in some organs. However, the amount by which this is achieved is uncertain and ill-understood (Nias, 1990)0 although, at the usually prescribed therapeutic doses (2500-6000cGy), the risk is believed to be much lower than that associated with lower doses given over a much longer period of time (Hilderley, 1992). Detailed discussions of radiation-induced carcinogenesis can be found in Bucholz (1990) and Nias (1990).

REFERENCES

Andersen BL, Tewfik HH, 1985, Psychological reactions to radiation therapy: reconsideration of the adaptive aspects of anxiety, Journal of Personal and Social Psychology, **48**, 1024-32.

Bucholz J, 1990, Radiation carcinogenesis. In: Hassey K, Hilderley L (Editors), Nursing Perspectives in Radiation Oncology, Delmar Publishers, New York.

Bushke F, Parker R, 1972, Radiation Therapy in Cancer Management, Grune and Stratton, New York.

Campbell I, Illingworth M, 1992, Can patients wash during radiotherapy to the breast or chest wall? A randomised controlled trial, Clinical Oncology **4**, 78-82.

Radiation-induced side-effects

Hilderley LJ, 1992, Radiotherapy. In: Groenwald SL, Frogge MH, Goodman M, Yarbro CH, (Editors), Treatment Modalities. Part III from Cancer Nursing: Principles and Practice (Second edition), Jones and Bartlett Publishers, Boston.

Kobashi-Schoot JAM, Hantwald GJFP, van Dam FSAM, Bruning PF 1985, Assessment of malaise in cancer patients treated with radiotherapy, Cancer Nursing, **8**, 306-313.

Nail LM, 1992, Fatigue. In: Groenwald SL, Frogge MH, Goodman M, Yarbro CH, (Editors), Treatment Modalities. Part III from Cancer Nursing: Principles and Practice (Second edition), Jones and Bartlett Publishers, Boston.

Nias AHW, 1988, Clinical Radiobiology (Second edition), Churchill Livingstone, Edinburgh.

Nias AHW, 1990, An Introduction to Radiobiology, John Wiley and Sons, Chichester.

Schnipper IM, 1985, Symptom management: Anorexia, Cancer Nursing, **8** (Suppl), 33-35.

Sutcliffe J, Holmes S, 1991, Quality of life: verification and use of a self-assessment scale in two patient populations, Journal of Advanced Nursing, **16**, 490-498.

Thomas S, 1990, Wound Management and Dressings, The Pharmaceutical Press, London.

CHAPTER 7   RADIOTHERAPY OF THE HEAD AND NECK

Radiation to the head and neck can result in a number of unpleasant side-effects that may significantly influence the patient's well-being through effects on his self-esteem and his ability to communicate. At the same time, oral complications may affect his ability to eat and drink thus compromising his nutritional status (Ch 14).

ALOPECIA
Since hair follicles undergo rapid cell division they are particularly sensitive to irradiation and hair loss is common. However, unlike that associated with cancer chemotherapy, alopecia occurs only in the area of the treatment field and may be transient or permanent depending on the dose of radiation administered.

During treatment of brain tumours or whole brain radiotherapy, alopecia follows a typical pattern. Gradual thinning of the hair will occur at a dose of about 2,500-3,000cGy. After 2-3 weeks, the remaining hair will fall out quite suddenly. In some cases, hair loss will be patchy. Here, hair loss affects the area(s) where radiation passes through the skull. Regrowth, where this occurs, usually begins within 2-3 months of treatment although the new hair may be of a different colour and texture.

Alopecia can be minimised by increasing the number and location of the radiation beams used in treatment. This is dependent on the site and histological type of tumour, the total dose of radiation and the dose:time relationship; it is, however, usual for more than one treatment field to be required to give an adequate tumour dose.

Care of the patient with alopecia
Alopecia can be traumatic having profound psychological effects on affected patients and the stress associated with both the anticipation and the experience of hair loss must not be overlooked. This possibility must be discussed with the patient before treatment starts so that appropriate measures can be planned to minimise changes in appearance.

Whether it involves head or body hair, the effect on the individual can be devastating, significantly altering their appearance and body image; considerable psychological support may be required. Understanding and support from both the caring team and the patient's 'significant others' is essential. Appropriate interventions include not only 'forewarning' the patient but discussing alternative courses of action and appropriate care.

When the treatment plan suggests that hair loss will be patchy the effect can be minimised if hair is kept long so that it can be arranged to cover affected areas. Care of the hair and scalp during therapy includes gentle brushing or combing and infrequent washing using a mild shampoo. Some radiotherapists prefer that patients do not wash their hair during the treatment period. Harsh chemicals (e.g. permanent waves, hair colours or bleach) are contraindicated since these may damage irradiated skin. Following washing, hair should be left to dry naturally since heated appliances should not be used.

When extensive hair loss is expected the patient may be advised to select a wig before this occurs. However, a wig may cause scalp irritation and some patients may prefer to wear a scarf, turban or hat to conceal hair loss. Of course, while a wig may improve a patient's outward appearance it will not compensate for the loss of hair although some patients can adapt to this with only minimal disruption.

CEREBRAL OEDEMA

When brain cells are included in the treatment field the resultant inflammatory response means that some degree of cerebral oedema is to be anticipated. This may exacerbate pre-existing neurological signs and symptoms or cause new signs and symptoms to develop (Table 7.1).

TABLE 7.1   Neurological signs and symptoms indicating raised intracranial pressure

---

Alterations in mental status - restlessness, irritability, confusion
Altered level of consciousness
Elevation of blood pressure
Gradual lowering of pulse and respiratory rate
Motor and sensory changes
Headache
Nausea - with/without projectile vomiting

NB.   Diagnosis is clinically difficult until overt signs and symptoms are present.

Cerebral oedema results in an increase in the water content of the brain leading to an increase in the tissue volume and, therefore, an increase in intracranial pressure. This, in turn, may be associated with an altered state of consciousness. As the oedema increases, cerebral blood flow is compromised and carbon dioxide is retained; blood vessels will dilate in an attempt to increase the availability of oxygen. This leads to a further increase in pressure and can lead to rapid deterioration in the patient's condition.

The patient should be warned that radiation may, in the short term, cause an increase in his symptoms. This should, however, be temporary and should improve once treatment is completed.

Corticosteroids, given 48-72 hours before the start of radiotherapy, are often used to reduce the incidence of radiation-induced cerebral oedema (Datz, 1986). Dexamethasone has been the drug of choice (Varrichio et al, 1992). Steroids should be given with food or milk and the concurrent administration of antacids is recommended to reduce the risk of gastrointestinal haemorrhage due to mucosal irritation.

When the condition is severe, osmotic diuretics, such as mannitol or urea, can be given to achieve cerebral decompression although their use is controversial as mannitol removes fluid from normal brain tissue and not from the oedematous tissue. Mannitol is, in addition, associated with a number of secondary problems including:

1. A 'rebound' effect in which, after an initial decrease, the intracranial pressure becomes high again
2. The production of a hyperosmolar state
3. Repeated use leads to decreased effectiveness
4. Aggravation of cerebral oedema in some patients.

(Youmans, 1973, Abels et al, 1986).

Hormones are occasionally given if, due to its location, the tumour has resulted in reduced production (Abels et al, 1986)

Care of the individual with cerebral oedema

Patient care centres on frequent, objective assessment followed by careful evaluation and detailed and accurate reporting (Table 7.2). Serial observations are valuable for comparison when new signs develop or changes occur. In simple terms, it is essential that nurses are constantly aware whether the patient is improving or his condition has remained unchanged or is showing signs of deterioration. Physicians are reliant on nurses for accurate reporting which will enable appropriate care to be rapidly initiated.

Table 7.2   Assessment of neurological function

Level of consciousness	Alert, lethargic, obtunded, stuporous, coma?
Mental status	Examples would include disordered behaviour or disorientation.
Respiratory pattern	Rate and depth of respiration, pattern changes, periods of apnoea, Cheyne-Stokes respiration, hyperventilation.
Pupil reactions	**a.** Responsiveness.
	b. Placement of eyes i. at rest
	ii. on stimulation.
Eye movements	Conjugate (do eyes move together)? Dysconjugate (deviation of one eye)?
Motor responses	Paresis or paralysis? Posture, reflexes.
Vital signs	Temperature, pulse, blood pressure.

Specific interventions are dependent on the underlying cause of the cerebral oedema and concurrent medical/surgical care.

Those patients receiving steroid therapy require close observation to ensure that steroid side-effects have not developed (Table 7.3). Should such effects arise, steroid doses are reduced immediately and 'tapered off' slowly to prevent the difficulties associated with rapid steroid withdrawal.

Table 7.3   Side-effects associated with steroid therapy

Acute adrenal insufficiency	Fatigue, muscular weakness, joint pain, fever, anorexia, nausea, orthostatic hypotension
Cardiovascular symptoms	Increased cardiac output, increased atrio-ventricular node conduction rate
Renal symptoms	Sodium retention
Gastrointestinal disturbances	Induction or aggravation of peptic ulcers, malaena leading to anaemia
Metabolic disturbances	Hyperglycaemia and glycosuria, polydipsia and polyuria
Musculoskeletal problems	Muscle atrophy, osteoporosis in those who are immobile, and pressure sores

Affected patients may require considerable reassurance and psychological support which must be continued until the cessation of treatment and the alleviation of neurological dysfunction. Care must be symptomatic and is designed to prevent further discomfort.

RADIATION-INDUCED CHANGES IN THE CENTRAL NERVOUS SYSTEM
Although the brain and spinal cord are believed to be relatively radio-resistant, radiation can, on occasions, cause a transient myelitis which affects both the upper and lower extremities and results in parathesiae and tingling. Since this does not arise for some time (1-12 months) after the completion of treatment these symptoms can be very disturbing for the patient and cause considerable concern and anxiety. Affected patients may require a great deal of support and reassurance that the symptoms usually improve gradually and spontaneously leaving no permanent effects; they do not indicate progression of the disease.

Rarely, radiation may result in permanent neurological damage. Occasionally, irreversible necrosis may follow cranial radiotherapy (Shewmon and Mosdeu, 1980). Such a reaction is not common but, when it does occur, may be indistinguishable from an extension of the neoplastic lesion.

ORAL COMPLICATIONS
The oral side-effects of radiotherapy to the head and neck can be extremely uncomfortable and distressing for the patient. It is important that the members of the caring team are familiar with the development, prevention and treatment of possible oral complications. The most common of these include:

- Mucositis/stomatitis
- Xerostomia
- Dental decay (caries)
- Hypersensitivity of the teeth
- Osteoradionecrosis.

Mucositis (stomatitis)
Stomatitis results from damage to the mucous membranes of the oral cavity. Since these membranes are continually subjected to considerable trauma, the cells are highly proliferative so as to replace those which are lost or damaged. Radiation, by inhibiting cellular replication, means that inadequate numbers of new cells are available to maintain mucosal integrity, the mucosa becomes thin and the signs and symptoms of mucositis appear.

83

Mucositis may be an acute or chronic reaction. It is an early sign of radiation injury arising after a dose of approximately 10Gy (Baker, 1982). In the early stages there will be mild erythema and possibly some loss of taste. The patient may complain of tenderness and, perhaps, some degree of xerostomia. The initial decrease in mitotic activity may lead to retention of superficial cells which, due to a greater degree of keratinisation, appear white. Radiation-induced leukoplakia is one of the earliest changes affecting the mouth. As these cells are shed, the mucosa becomes denuded and friable. As the total dose reaches 25Gy, oedema becomes more noticeable as the erythema diminishes due to pressure on the capillaries which causes stretching of the mucous membranes and breakdown of the oral tissues.

Cell death and inhibited mitosis, together with continuing surface cell loss, exacerbate discomfort causing pain and progressive mucosal atrophy; even minor trauma may cause painful erosions and ulceration predisposing to secondary, opportunistic infection so that the importance of oral hygiene cannot be over-emphasised. After 30Gy, the tongue may become swollen or ulcerated; both eating and talking become uncomfortable. Increased permeability, in both blood vessels and extravascular tissue, leads to oedema of the connective tissue thus increasing local breakdown.

By the completion of treatment, oral reactions reach their maximum. A fibrous exudate may cover affected areas creating a glistening white or yellow 'pseudomembrane' (radioepithelite) (Leahy et al, 1979) which is confluent over the radiated tissue and which is similar to that formed in the presence of infection with *Candida albicans* (thrush) (McGaw and Main, 1983). This is due to the extravasation of plasma from damaged capillaries and an accumulation of dead cells on the radiated surface. The radioepithelite should not be removed since the underlying epithelial surface is denuded and haemorrhage is likely (Baker, 1982). However, even minor trauma may disturb the membranes so that ulceration develops (Dudjak, 1987). Mucositis is a self-limiting symptom that usually resolves 2-4 weeks after treatment although, due to vascular and connective tissue damage, recovery is seldom complete (Baker, 1982)

Mucositis is exacerbated when nutritional status is poor, particularly when there are deficiencies of the B complex vitamins (especially folic acid, riboflavin (B_2) and cyanocobalamin (B_{12})), zinc and vitamin C. Other factors causing dryness and/or trauma to the mucous membranes, such as oxygen therapy, mouth breathing, dehydration and poor oral hygiene, may all contribute to an exacerbation so that care must be taken to minimise their effects.

Even when recovery from an acute reaction has taken place there may still be some important late changes due primarily to damage to the microcirculation and supporting tissues. These may result in hypotrophic mucous membranes which are hypersensitive and slow to recover from even minor trauma so that any minor surgical procedure (e.g. dental extraction) carries an increased risk of infection or chronic ulceration.

Care of the patient with mucositis/stomatitis

Successful care is often dependent on teaching the patient to identify and manage those factors which may prevent complications and maintain comfort. To this end, there are many similarities between the management of mucositis and that of xerostomia.

When mucositis is an anticipated effect of treatment, the oral cavity should be regularly assessed noting areas of dryness, inflammation, ulceration or other breaks in the mucosal integrity and the presence of radioepithelite and/or infection so that appropriate care can be instigated. Since systemic infection often originates from the mouth (McElroy, 1984), temperature should be monitored four hourly and swabs taken for bacterial culture from any lesion or when an infection is suspected.

Regular oral care must be carried out to promote and maintain a satisfactory state of health in the tissues and secretions of the oral cavity. Its purpose is therefore:

- Prevention of infection, periodontal disease and gingival bleeding
- Improvement of general well-being
- Prevention of further damage to oral structure
- Reduction of oral complications so that treatment can be completed

(Daeffler, 1980; Johnson and Gross, 1985).

Although a number of measures can be used to treat stomatitis, it is important to enlist the patient's help in achieving this. He should be advised to avoid irritant substances, such as alcohol, tobacco and hot spicy or acid foods; very cold foods may also be irritant. He should also be advised to avoid commercial mouthwashes which are astringent, even when diluted, and may potentiate oral damage.

When patient is psychologically dependant on alcohol or tobacco, which are often used to relieve stress and anxiety, considerable empathy and understanding will be needed.

The teeth must be gently but carefully brushed using a soft toothbrush, after every meal and at bedtime. The Bass technique of brushing has been suggested to be 'the best at meeting the requirement of proper oral hygiene and is relatively simple for the patient to learn' (Trowbridge and Carl, 1975). This technique involves use of a small, soft toothbrush which is placed at a 45° angle between the gingiva and the teeth and moved in short, horizontal strokes. The lingual surfaces of both the upper and lower anterior teeth are cleaned using the tip or heel of the toothbrush (Dudjak, 1987).

The mouth should be regularly rinsed using warm saline solutions or non-alcohol containing mouthwashes, such as 0.5% chlorhexidine in water (1ml chlorhexidine in 200ml water) since alcohol will enhance dryness and cause desiccation of the membranes. This means that the commonly used glycerine (glycerol) and lemon swabs should also be avoided. In fact, as long ago as 1969, Wiley suggested that glycerol and lemon were neither acceptable cleansers nor effective oral care agents.

Commercial mouthwashes containing detergents should also be avoided as detergent removes mucins from the tissues. In general, it is believed that it is the frequency and regularity of oral care that improves the condition of the mouth rather than the specific agent involved (Dudjak, 1987). Since the basic value of any mouthwash depends on its mechanical actions in washing away loose debris as well as its physical action of moistening and softening the oral mucosa, normal saline and glycothymoline will be effective mouthwashes and also leave subjective feelings of freshness and temporary relief of xerostomia (Daeffler, 1980).

Thorough but gentle mouth irrigation can be soothing and will help to decrease the risk of infection by loosening retained food particles and breaking up tenacious mucus. Regular brushing of the teeth using a soft toothbrush, foam sticks or cotton buds is recommended when this can be tolerated. The mouth must be cleaned every 2-4 hours using normal saline or other mild mouthwash. Although hydrogen peroxide has been used in the care of mucositis for many years, this can damage oral tissues if it is not diluted appropriately. A 1:1 solution can, however, be helpful; the lips can be kept moist using pure lanolin or other lip salve.

Trauma to the membranes must be avoided. Loose dentures, for example, cause friction to the gums and provide a food trap so that, unless they can be adapted or relined, dentures are best worn only when necessary (e.g. when eating). Regular analgesia may be needed both to promote comfort and to ensure an adequate food intake. Topical anaesthetics, such as lignocaine hydrochloride, prior to meals may also enhance the ability to eat although some people find their anaesthetic properties objectionable particularly on the tongue. They may also adversely affect taste sensation further inhibiting food consumption. Adequate nutrition is essential if cellular repair and regeneration are to occur. Dietary manipulation, including nutritious but soft and bland foods, is essential (see Ch 14).

Xerostomia

Since the salivary glands are highly sensitive to radiation (Carl, 1983) radiotherapy will destroy their function, especially if the parotid glands have been irradiated, thus altering salivary flow to the mouth. After a dose of about 10Gy, the saliva begins to change progressing from a thin watery fluid to a thick viscous fluid of a ropey consistency which loses its lubricating qualities and adheres to the mucosa and teeth. This makes eating, swallowing and chewing difficult and may also interfere with chemical digestion and taste sensation (Navazesh and Ship, 1983); it may also make both talking and oral hygiene difficult and painful. Such effects may be a permanent effect of treatment since recovery is rare; even when xerostomia is temporary it may take 6-12 months for recovery to occur (Baker, 1982).

Xerostomia has been associated with many complications including increased dental caries and periodontal disease, mucositis, disturbed oral sensations and changes in taste sensation (e.g. Ross and Holbrook, 1984) so that this may exacerbate the difficulties associated with radiation therapy. Dryness of the mouth can be distressing and its effects cannot be overemphasised; appropriate care is, therefore, vital to patient comfort and quality of life as well as in the prevention of additional complications.

Care of the xerostomic patient

The patient should be taught to adopt measures that will help to maintain the moisture of the mucous membranes, maintain, or enhance, oral protective mechanisms, and avoid trauma to the membranes. An increased consumption of fluids, preferably water, sipped at frequent intervals throughout the day, highly flavoured lozenges and sugar-free chewing gum may help to keep the membranes moist. The patient should be advised to avoid sugar, and sugar-containing products, as the combination of xerostomia and sucrose is likely to enhance the development of dental caries.

As normal saliva plays an important role in controlling the balance of the oral flora its absence significantly increases the risk of infection since this promotes the development of microbial plaque and the emergence of a highly cariogenic microflora (Brown et al, 1975). This explains the increased incidence of *Candida albicans*, and other infections, seen in xerostomic patients and stresses the need for a regular and effective mouth care regime.

Mouthwashes, such as normal saline or glycothymoline, may provide moisture leaving subjective feelings of freshness and temporarily relieve xerostomia. Artificial saliva can be used to supplement the reduced production of both mucous and serious secretions and several commercial products are available. However, the sensitivity of the oral mucosa may preclude their use in some patients. When appropriate, saliva substitutes should be used as often as is necessary to maintain comfort although the volume used should be the minimum required to maintain internal lubrication (Navazesh and Ship, 1983). Excessive quantities of artificial saliva simply serve to enhance discomfort. 1-2ml will often maintain lubrication for as long as 12hrs. Pure lanolin, Vaseline or other lip salves can be applied to keep the lips moist.

Dental decay

Radiation-induced dental decay has long been a recognised hazard of this mode of treatment (e.g. Trowbridge and Carl, 1975). Although it usually arises some time after treatment, appropriate care during therapy can greatly reduce its occurrence. The reduced volume and altered composition of the saliva, alterations in the oral microflora, reduced lubrication and soft food tend to result in stagnation of the oral secretions and food remnants causing debris to cling to the teeth and engendering widespread caries. At the same time, changes in the salivary pH affect its buffering capacity (Ross and Holbrook, 1984). As the pH decreases demineralisation of the enamel accelerates (Marsh and Martin, 1984) particularly as the acidic saliva tends to pool at the gingival margin encouraging the characteristic pattern of caries seen in irradiated patients. Decay is shallow but tends to extend around the neck of the tooth so that it is not unusual for caries to cause amputation of the teeth at the gingival margin (McGaw and Main, 1983).

Oral hygiene is vital to the prevention of radiation-induced damage to the teeth and brushing the teeth with a soft bristled brush several times daily is recommended. The topical application of fluoride may be valuable and fluoride is available in a variety of mouthwashes, topical solutions and toothpastes. Dental examination is essential before treatment commences and teeth showing evidence of decay may have to be extracted. Extractions, and other dental treatment, must be carried out 10-14 days prior to radiotherapy to allow healing to take place (Lane and Forgay, 1981; Westcott, 1985).

At the same time, hypersensitivity of the teeth may occur affecting, primarily, the cervical area of the teeth even in the absence of any decay. This is believed to be due to denaturation of the organic components of the tooth. Such hypersensitivity, particularly when combined with mucositis, may indirectly contribute to an increased incidence of dental decay as the patient may be reluctant to brush his teeth due to the discomfort and pain this will cause. Overcoming these problems requires considerable skill and tact and support and encouragement are essential to ensure the continuation of effective oral care throughout treatment.

OSTEORADIONECROSIS

The high density of bone can result in delivery of a high dose of radiation to its cellular components although the use of super- and megavoltage machines has led to a reduction in both bone and vascular damage. However, extension of caries into the dental pulp, and the spread of infection to the periapical tissues, may transfer infection to the bone thus causing osteoradionecrosis (ORN).

All patients who have received radiation to the head and neck are susceptible to ORN which may occur several months or years after completion of treatment (Levin and Ferris, 1980). Poor oral hygiene and continued use of oral irritants (e.g. alcohol, tobacco) are major contributory factors. ORN is a progressive and irreversible condition that more commonly affects the mandible than the maxilla. This is because the blood supply to the mandible is less profuse than that to the maxilla (Westcott, 1985). Its effects are that the bone marrow becomes cellular and avascular and displays fatty degeneration and increased fibrosis so that the bone is unable to respond to trauma or infection (Beumer et al, 1979). Such changes are subclinical and cannot be detected by either patient or clinician. However, as ORN progresses, the patient will suffer severe pain, chronic mucosal ulceration and osteomyelitis (Morrish, 1981; Carl, 1983).

The presence of carious teeth, other oral or systemic infection or xerostomia will greatly increase the risk of ORN that tends to occur in those with chronic and advanced periodontal disease (Carl 1983). This serves to emphasise, yet again, the need for meticulous oral hygiene and the need to maintain healthy teeth by means of a comprehensive fluoridation programme (Ritchie et al, 1985). If ORN develops it should be managed with irrigation, gentle debridement and good oral hygiene; antibiotic therapy will be prescribed. If ORN is treated surgically this often creates extensive necrosis; conservative management will promote healing in the majority of cases.

LATE EFFECTS OF RADIATION

The late effects of radiotherapy can result in motor disturbances of the trigeminal nerve, especially spasm or inflammation of the masticatory muscles, and an associated difficulty in opening the mouth (Miller et al, 1981). Optimal function must be maintained so that mouth exercises may be recommended and the use of oral prostheses and appliances may be required to prevent closure and extension of the defect.

PHARYNGITIS

Depending on the area of the treatment field, mucositis may extend to include the pharynx and the oesophagus causing extreme discomfort. Since oesophagitis is more common in patients under-going treatment to the area of the chest and thorax this is discussed in Ch 8.

Pharyngitis may occur approximately 2 weeks after the start of treatment and persist for 2-4 weeks after its completion; on occasions it may be so severe as to necessitate discontinuation of the treatment to allow healing to take place.

Pharyngitis is manifested by a sore throat, an irritant, hacking cough and varying degrees of dysphagia. These symptoms may significantly affect food and fluid intake and influence the patient's willingness and/or ability to talk due to the discomfort this causes.

Treatment includes rest, a liquid or soft diet, aspirin or other analgesic agent and warm saline gargles. Alternatively throat irrigation may be more effective since gargling will not reach all parts of the pharynx and may also increase discomfort by stretching the inflamed tissue producing tension and pain. This is achieved by attaching a rubber tube, to which an irrigating tip is attached, to an irrigation can filled with the desired irrigating solution at the appropriate temperature. This is then hung above the patient's head while the patient leans over a collecting basin so that fluid will run back out of the mouth. The nozzle is inserted into the mouth, without touching the base of the tongue or uvula (as this will cause gagging), and, while holding the breath to prevent aspiration, the patient directs the solution so that all parts of the throat are irrigated. It is necessary to clamp the tubing at intervals to enable the patient to breathe and rest since 1-2 litres of fluid are used. The irrigating solution may be normal saline, sodium bicarbonate or a mild anti-septic; sodium bicarbonate is particularly effective when secretions are tenacious. Solutions are used as hot as the patient can tolerate although they should never be hotter than 120°F (48.8°C).

Both gargling and throat irrigations are soothing and will aid patient comfort. They will help to loosen and remove secretions and, by causing local vasodilation, will increase the surface blood supply. Local anaesthetics and antiseptics may also be applied by means of a throat spray.

Oral hygiene and mouth care form an important part of care and are refreshing for the patient so helping to maintain his comfort. This will also help to prevent drying and cracking of the lips and reduce the risk of secondary oral infection. Antitussive agents may be prescribed for the relief of the patient's cough.

TASTE ABERRATION

Taste changes are common during radiation to the head and neck, particularly when the tongue is included in the treatment field. Such changes may persist even after completion of therapy. They are primarily due to damage to the taste buds together with salivary changes although it must be recognised that taste changes may arise in any patient with cancer (e.g. Holmes and Dickerson, 1988).

The majority of the four primary taste receptors (bitter, sweet, salt and sour) are located on the tongue although taste buds are also present on the palate, tonsillar pillars and nasopharynx. These combine to give hundreds of different taste sensations which are detected and integrated by the nervous system.

Taste changes, which may arise within 2 weeks of the start of treatment, show no uniform pattern although alterations in sweet and bitter thresholds are the most common (Calman, 1982). This means, for example, an elevation in the sucrose (sweet) recognition threshold or a lowered urea (bitter) recognition threshold. A decreased response to sweet tastes means that food or drinks must be sweeter if they are to be recognised as sweet. A lowered bitter threshold may be manifested by an aversion to red meat. However, changes may affect any of the primary taste sensations and some patients experience a general loss of taste which has been termed 'mouth blindness' (MacCarthy-Leventhal, 1959). Some patients develop unpleasant tastes. For example, a burnt taste may be evident; affected patients may find the taste of coffee and chocolate, for example, very unpleasant (Iwamoto, 1992) As a result, each patient must be individually assessed and it is not possible to suggest any single way in which the problem can be overcome. Limited evidence suggests that improvement may follow an objective response to treatment (Lowe, 1986), although some changes may be permanent. Recovery from xerostomia may play an important part in regaining normal taste sensation.

LEARNED FOOD AVERSION

Taste aberrations are important not only because of their contribution to anorexia but also for their possible role in the development of food aversions which are not uncommon in cancer patients. Such aversions may also arise as a learned response to the association between symptoms and the disease or its treatment (Bernstein and Bernstein, 1981; Leathwood et al, 1986). This effect is regarded as a variant of classical conditioning in which a conditioned stimulus (i.e. taste) becomes associated with an unconditioned response (e.g. discomfort) (Bolles, 1975). Animal studies have shown that just one pairing of a food with GI discomfort induced by radiotherapy is sufficient to cause continued avoidance of that food even after treatment has been completed. Such effects appear to cause aversion to even the most novel food(s) consumed around the time discomfort is experienced (Revusky and Bedarf, 1967) and this has been used to good effect in developing approaches to overcoming this problem.

For example, Broberg and Bernstein (1987) have shown that using 'scapegoats' can reduce the impact of food aversion on normal food items. Using this approach, foods that are not important in the normal diet (e.g. sweets) are introduced just before therapy begins the theory being that an aversion to such items will have little or no impact on nutrient consumption. Mattes et al (1987) have shown that this is effective in treating adults receiving chemotherapy; it may also prove to be beneficial to those undergoing radiotherapy.

Care of the patient with taste changes or food aversion

Care can only be prescribed on an individual basis. Dietary modification and avoidance of disliked food(s) will usually overcome food aversion. When the condition is severe, and diet very restricted, advice may be required from a dietician or nurse-nutritionist. Appropriate care is directed towards overcoming the effects of taste aberration so as to maintain an adequate food and fluid intake.

Since evidence suggests a relationship between trace mineral deficiencies, particularly zinc deficiency, and taste aberration (Hambidge et al, 1972) it is possible that zinc supplementation may help to overcome hypoguesia (diminished taste) and dysguesia (loss of taste) in some patients. This is not, however, likely to be beneficial when the changes are due to radiation-induced destruction of the taste buds.

Since taste changes are highly variable each patient must be assessed on an individual basis so as to identify those factors that may be contributory to taste change and that may, in turn, decrease food intake. Changes in the taste of 'normal' foods may significantly alter the usual eating pattern causing distress to the patient, who can no longer enjoy his favourite foods, and stress for the carer who may find it difficult to persuade him to eat.

It is, therefore, important that both the patient and his family understand that this is the consequence of the disease and/or its treatment. The patient must be persuaded to eat and this is best achieved by giving consideration to the identification of a variety of acceptable foods and planning the diet with these in mind.

Clearly the presence and degree of taste alteration must be assessed. Common complaints include:

- A decrease in the sensation of sweet tastes so that additional sugar is necessary for this taste to be recognised. This can be beneficial in those patients requiring a high energy intake (see Ch. 14)

93

- Conversely, there may be an increased recognition of sweet tastes so that care must be taken to ensure that the patient is not given foods/drinks which are too sweet
- Changes in the recognition of bitter tastes may occur which pose particular problems when protein-containing foods are consumed. Beef and pork are the foods most commonly rejected although any protein food (e.g. fish, eggs and poultry) may be affected. Other foods, such as those which are naturally sour or bitter (e.g. tomatoes, lemons and other citrus fruit, coffee, tea and chocolate) may also be rejected (see Holmes, 1993)
- On occasions the patient may complain of a persistent metallic taste that is not related to any specific food. This is, perhaps, the most difficult to overcome. Clearly, canned products should be avoided and the use of plastic cutlery may be helpful. Other unpleasant tastes must be treated on a symptomatic basis
- Hypoguesia or dysguesia may lead to a condition referred to as 'mouth blindness' (MacCarthy-Leventhal, 1959) when all food is described as tasting like 'cotton wool' or 'chalk'. Since both these substances are difficult to chew and swallow the inevitable difficulty in eating can have a major effect on the patient's food intake.

All these effects may have a significant impact on the patient's nutritional status so that regular assessment is an essential part of care (Ch 14).

Appropriate interventions

Once the occurrence of taste changes has been recognised and affected foods identified, it should prove to be relatively straight-forward to plan an appropriate diet which excludes foods for which the patient has expressed a dislike or aversion. Alternatively, spices, herbs and other flavouring agents (such as onions, garlic, and fruit juices) can be added to foods/dishes in an attempt to mask the taste changes. This can be difficult to achieve, particularly in the hospital setting, and it can take a considerable amount of ingenuity before successful solutions are identified for individual patients.

However difficult, it is important that the patient is persuaded to eat since it is vital that nutritional status is maintained; this may have a significant impact on the quality of the patient's life (Holmes,

1986). Alternative approaches can be tried to tempt the patient to consume an adequate diet.

- Serve foods hot/warm as this will help to intensify the taste
- Ensure that food smells 'good' and looks attractive since the odour and appearance of food plays a major role in stimulating the appetite and tempting the patient to eat
- Ensure that foods are moist and easy to eat. Add sauces, gravies and dressings to meals or, alternatively, use an artificial saliva to increase the amount of moisture in the mouth as food must be in solution before it can be tasted. Do not, however, encourage fluids to be taken with meals as this promotes satiety and may limit the amount of food consumed
- Provide small, nutrient dense meals or snacks at frequent intervals (for example 6 times a day) since small amounts may be better tolerated. Large amounts of food may be very off putting to some patients
- Ensure that any liquids taken are nutritious such as fruit juices or milk drinks
- The patient should be taught the importance of food. This should be regarded as an important part of treatment and can, if necessary, be regarded as a form of 'medicine' that must be taken regularly.

Since taste alteration may be a permanent consequence of radio-therapy, and since cancer is rarely an acutely fatal disease (Shils, 1977), this may become a chronic disability. As a result it is vital that the patient is helped to come to terms with this and taught how best to overcome its effects and maintain his food intake.

EFFECTS OF RADIATION ON THE EYE

Radiation may cause both acute and late effects when the eye is included in the treatment field so that, whenever possible, the eye is protected by means of lead shielding. Conjunctivitis and keratitis may develop as acute effects when the total dose received reaches 2,500-3,000cGy. Similarly, lacrimal gland secretion may be inhibited.

Late effects may include lenticular opacities and the development of cataracts; corneal ulceration and glaucoma may also occur (Strohl, 1988). Opacities/cataracts that interfere with vision may require surgical intervention. As a result, patients who have received radio-therapy to a field which includes the eye should undergo regular visual assessment and examination of the eyes to determine the extent of visual impairment; trauma to the eye should be avoided and patients should be advised to avoid rubbing or over-wiping the eyes. Handkerchiefs should not be used but replaced with tissues that can be discarded after use. Sun glasses may provide protection.

REFERENCES

Abels L, Belcher A, Russo BL, 1986, The nervous system. In: Abels L (Editor), Critical Care Nursing: A Physiological Approach, CV Mosby, St Louis.

Baker DG, 1982, The radiobiological basis for tissue reactions in the oral cavity following therapeutic X-irradiation, Archives of Otolaryngology, **108**, 21-29.

Bernstein IL, Bernstein ID, 1981, Learned food aversions and cancer anorexia, Cancer Treatment Reports, **65**, (suppl), 43-47.

Beumer J, Curtis T, Harrison RE, 1979, Radiation therapy of the oral cavity: sequelae and management, Part 1, Head and Neck Surgery, **1**, 301-312.

Bolles RC, 1975, Learning Theory, Rhinehart and Wilson, New York.

Broberg DJ, Bernstein L, 1987, Candy as a scapegoat in the prevention of food aversion in children receiving chemotherapy, Cancer, **60**, 2344-2347.

Brown L, Dreizen S, Handler S, Johnston D, 1975, Effect of radiation-induced xerostomia on human oral microflora, Journal of Dental Research, **54**, 740-749.

Calman KC, 1982, Cancer cachexia, British Journal of Hospital Medicine, **27**, 28-34.

Carl W, 1974, Oral and dental care for the irradiated patient, Periodontics and Oral Hygiene, **10**, 55-62.

Carl W, 1983. Oral complications in cancer patients, American Family Physician, **27**, 161-170.

Daeffler R, 1980, Oral hygiene measures for patients with cancer, Cancer Nursing, **3**, 347-356.

Datz FL, 1986, Cerebral Oedema following iodine-131 therapy for thyroid carcinoma metastasic to the brain, Journal of Nuclear Medicine, **27**, 637-640.

Dudjak LA, 1987, Mouth care for mucositis due to radiation therapy, Cancer Nursing, **10**, 131-140.

Hambidge KM, Hambidge C, Jacobs M, Baum JD, 1972, Low levels of zinc in hair, anorexia, poor growth and hypoguesia in children,

Paediatric Research, **6**, 868-876.

Holmes S, 1993, Food avoidance in patients undergoing chemo-therapy, Supportive Care in Cancer, **1**, 326-330.

Holmes S, Dickerson JWT, 1988, Malignant disease: nutritional implications of disease and treatment, Cancer and Metastasis Reviews **6**, 357-381

Iwamoto RR, 1992, Alterations in oral status. In: Groenwald SL, Frogge MH. Goodman M, Yarbro CH, (Editors), Manifestations of Cancer and Cancer Treatments. Part V from Cancer Nursing: Principles and Practice, Jones and Bartlett Publishers, Boston.

Johnson BL, Gross J, 1985, Handbook of Oncology Nursing, John Wiley and Sons, New York.

Lane B, Forgay M, 1981, Upgrading your oral hygiene protocol for the patient with cancer, Cancer Nursing, **7**, 27-29.

Leahy D, St Germain J, Varrichio C, 1979, The Nurse and Radiotherapy, C V Mosby, St Louis.

Leathwood PD, Ashley DV, Moennoz DV, 1986, Anorexia and cachexia in cancer, Nestlé Research News 1985/86, Nestec, Switzerland.

Levin AC, Ferris GM, 1980, The treatment of post-radiation therapy patients, Florida Dental Journal, **51**, 41-44.

Lowe O, 1986, Pretreatment dental assessment and management of patients undergoing head and neck irradiation, Clinical Preventive Dentistry, **8**, 24-30.

MacCarthy-Leventhal EM, 1959, Post-radiation mouth blindness, Lancet **ii** 1138-1139.

Marsh P, Martin M, 1984, Oral microbiology (Second edition) Van Nostrand Reinhold (UK) Co. Ltd., Berkshire.

Mattes RD, Arnold C, Boraas M, 1987, Management of learned food aversions in cancer patients receiving chemotherapy, Cancer Treatment Reports, **71**, 1071-1078.

McElroy TH, 1984, Infection in the patient receiving chemotherapy for cancer: oral considerations, Journal of the American Dental Association, **109**, 454-456.

McGaw W, Main J, 1983, Dental care for cancer patients, Journal of the Canadian Dental Association, **6**, 417-423.

Miller EC, Vergo TJ, Feldman MI, 1981, Dental management of patients undergoing radiation therapy for cancer of the head and neck, The Compendium of Continuing Education, **2**, 350-356.

Morrish R, 1981, Osteo-radio-necrosis in patients irradiated for head and neck carcinoma, Cancer, **47**, 1980-1982.

Navazesh M, Ship II, 1983, Xerostomia: diagnosis and treatment, American Journal of Otolaryngology, **4**, 283-292.

Ritchie JR, Brown JR, Guerra RA, Klimek JJ, Nightingale CH, 1984, Dental care for the irradiated patient, Quintessence International, **16**, 837-842.

Revusky SH, Bedarf EW, 1967, Association of illness with prior ingestion of novel foods, Science, **155**, 219-220.

Ross P, Holbrook W, 1984, Clinical and Oral Microbiology, Blackwell Scientific Publications, Oxford.

Shewmon DA, Mosdeu JC, 1980, Delayed radiation necrosis of the brain contralateral to original tumour, Archives of Neurology, **37**, 592-593.

Shils ME, 1977, Nutritional problems induced by cancer, Medical Clinics of North America, **63**, 1009-1025.

Strohl R, 1988, The nursing role in radiation oncology. Symptom management of acute and chronic reactions, Oncology Nursing Forum, **15**, 429-434.

Trowbridge J, Carl W, 1975, Oral care of the patient having head and neck irradiation, American Journal of Nursing, **75**, 2146-2149.

Varrichio CG, Miller N, Pazdur M, 1992, Edema and effusions. In: Groenwald SL, Frogge MH. Goodman M, Yarbro CH, (Editors), Manifestations of Cancer and Cancer Treatments. Part V from Cancer Nursing: Principles and Practice, Jones and Bartlett Publishers, Boston.

Westcott WB, 1985, Dental management of patients being treated for oral cancer, CDA Journal, **13**,42-47.

Wiley S, 1969, Why glycerol and lemon juice? American Journal of Nursing, **69**, 343-344.

Youmans J, 1973 (Editor), Neurological Surgery, Volumes 1, 2 and 3, WB Saunders Co., Philadelphia.

CHAPTER 8   RADIATION TO THE CHEST AND THORAX

Radiation directed towards any area of the chest and thorax may cause unpleasant and disturbing side-effects some of which may indicate that radiation tolerance has been exceeded and may necessitate discontinuation of therapy. The late effects may lead to a permanent reduction in pulmonary function and an increased susceptibility to infection.

OESOPHAGITIS

Since the mucosa of the oesophagus is continuous with that of the oral epithelium it too is vulnerable to radiation-induced damage. Oesophagitis may arise when an area of the oesophagus is included in the treatment field. It results from the effects of radiation on the rapidly dividing mucosal cells causing oedema and inflammation and, in severe cases, ulceration which may be so severe as to necessitate that treatment is discontinued to allow healing to take place. It can cause significant pain and, even when it is not severe, oesophagitis may be extremely uncomfortable and can significantly limit food/fluid intake. The clinical symptoms may range from mild substernal burning to severe dysphagia accompanied by severe angina-like chest pain which is usually triggered by swallowing (Finkelstein, 1986).

Oesophagitis usually arises 2-3 weeks after the start of treatment, after a dose of 2000-3000cGy, and subsides several weeks after treatment is completed. In view of the severity and degree of discomfort caused by oesophagitis it is usual for the oesophagus to be shielded during treatment if it is included in the radiation field but is not involved with the tumour itself.

The incidence and severity of oesophagitis increases with increasing doses of radiation. The risk is exacerbated by the presence of cancer of the oesophagus, the total dose of radiation delivered and concurrent chemotherapy (Unsawasdi et al, 1985; Stevens, 1989). The oesophagus can, in general, withstand doses of radiation of up to 6500cGy over a period of 6-7 weeks (Stevens, 1989); a dose of 7500cGy increases the likelihood of ulceration or stricture some years after the completion of therapy.

Oesophagitis is manifested by:

- Sore throat
- Sensation of a 'lump' in the throat

99

- Difficulty in swallowing, particularly solid foods (dysphagia)
- Burning or substernal pain
- Pain on swallowing.

It may be accompanied by a severe and constant substernal pain which closely resembles that associated with myocardial infarction; this must be excluded before the diagnosis is confirmed. Once oesophagitis is confirmed the goals of care become:

1. Alleviation/minimisation of pain and discomfort.
2. Provision of optimal nutritional and fluid replacement.

Care of the patient with oesophagitis

The aim of care is to prevent further irritation of the oesophageal mucosa. Treatment is largely symptomatic and supportive; the patient should be warned of the possibility that oesophagitis may arise.

In the acute phase, a liquid diet is advised as this is less abrasive to the inflamed area. When solids can be tolerated, foods given should be bland and soothing and small frequent meals will help to prevent gastric distension and reduce gastric acid secretion. Gastric reflux must be prevented and the irritating ability of the gastric juices decreased. Antacids will help to reduce gastric acidity and Gaviscon™, a mixture of alginic acid and aluminium hydroxide - is a useful adjunct to treatment since this floats on the surface of the gastric acid pool reducing the movement of acid into the oesophagus. Although milk and milk products can be soothing, high protein foods should generally be avoided during the acute phase of an oesophageal reaction since protein will stimulate gastrin production and increase pressure on the lower oesophageal sphincter thus increasing the risk of gastric reflux.

Bland foods that are soft and smooth will be easier for the patient to swallow and the addition of gravy or sauces can be helpful. Foods that are chemically, mechanically or thermally irritating should be avoided. Thus, hot or spicy foods are best avoided and cold foods or foods served at room temperature are recommended. The patient may find alcoholic or carbonated drinks irritating and acidic foods, such as citrus fruit or fruit juices, uncomfortable. Dry or hard foods, such as biscuits and raw foods and vegetables, may be difficult to swallow. However, as each patient is an individual he will identify those foods that are most acceptable and may find food brought in from home more appealing than mass produced, hospital catering. Since these patients are at considerable nutritional risk this practice should be encouraged where appropriate. Foods offered should be high in calories and provide adequate amounts of protein and other nutrients. A liquid nutritional supplement (see Ch 14) may be an appropriate adjunct to treatment when food intake is severely restricted; alternatively tube feeding or total parenteral nutrition may be required. Such patients may require nutritional counselling.

Systemic analgesics, prior to meals, may provide general relief from oesophageal pain; liquid preparations such as Mucaine™ or aspirin solutions, may provide local relief. Nifedipine, an antispasmodic agent, has been reported to be effective in relieving radiation-induced oesophagitis by reducing oesophageal spasm (Unsawasdi et al, 1985).

Because the gag reflex may be decreased, a nurse or family member should always be present when the patient is eating so that swift action can be initiated should complications result. Certain general measures will, however, be valuable when caring for the dysphagic patient. These include:

1. Elevation of the head of the bed to reduce the risk of regurgitation and inhalation of the gastric content.
2. To reduce the risk of regurgitation still further, no food should be taken within 2-3 hours of going to bed.
3. Provision of a high energy (calorie), moderate protein pureed or liquid diet which provides for all nutrient requirements including the trace nutrients (minerals and vitamins).
4. Stagnating oesophageal content should, where necessary, be removed by careful lavage using a wide bore tube. This is necessary to prevent inhalation during sleep, to reduce mucosal inflammation and to improve swallowing. Great care is required in carrying out this procedure to avoid further damage to the oesophageal mucosa.

Once the acute phase has subsided, a high energy, high protein diet is essential to promote recovery and cellular regeneration. It cannot be stressed highly enough that the maintenance of hydration and an adequate diet are of paramount importance in the care of any affected patient. The late effects of radiation may result in strictures and stenosis (due to fibrosis) leading to obstruction; ulceration and oesophageal perforation may also develop although these are, more commonly, due to local tumour necrosis (Stevens, 1989). Periodic oesophageal dilatation may be needed to widen the oesophagus and permit swallowing. Affected patients may require nutritional advice to enable them to modify their diet appropriately. High calorie, high carbohydrate and protein liquid supplements may be needed. Soft, pureed or liquidised foods from the patient's usual diet may be tried. Alternatively, nasogastric or ostomy feeding may be required to ensure provision of an adequate nutrient intake (see Ch 14).

EFFECTS ON THE HEART

Cardiac side-effects may arise if the heart or its vasculature are included in the treatment field. Blood vessels may become occluded when radiation-induced damage affects the endothelium. Thrombosis may occur. Although the heart muscle itself is relatively radio-resistant an acute but transient pericarditis may occur at doses above 4000cGy (Strohl, 1988).

Pericarditis and myocarditis may, occasionally, arise some years after radiotherapy; fibrosis and an increased risk of coronary artery disease may also be present. As a result, cardiac function should be regularly evaluated including assessment of chest pain (often of a pleuritic nature), tachycardia and electrocardiogram abnormalities.

Care and treatment includes analgesic relief of pain, often based on aspirin, and, occasionally, corticosteroid therapy to reduce inflammation. The patient must be observed carefully for complications such as cardiac tamponade (Ch 13). Restrictions on activity may vary from bed rest in the acute stage to gradually increasing periods out of bed as symptoms abate. On occasions the patient is able to remain active for as long as his heart is able to compensate although his activity may be limited by reduced cardiac efficiency.

INDIGESTION, NAUSEA AND VOMITING

Although not common accompaniments to radiotherapy, indigestion, nausea and vomiting are unpleasant and distressing symptoms that may cause the patient considerable discomfort. Vomiting is, in any case, generally less severe than that associated with cancer chemotherapy. There are similarities between these symptoms so that it is convenient for them to be considered together.

Indigestion is the term used to describe a feeling of discomfort in the epigastric region or the back of the throat. It may be accompanied by heartburn, regurgitation of the acidic gastric contents, belching, distension and/or nausea. Nausea describes a feeling of discomfort, again in the epigastric region, which frequently occurs in a wave-like fashion and is often accompanied by the need to vomit. As a result, it usually precedes vomiting. Vomiting is a somatic response involving forceful ejection of the stomach contents or, on occasions, those of the duodenum and jejunum, through the oral cavity usually, but not exclusively, preceded by nausea and hypersalivation.

Nausea and vomiting may be accompanied by a wide range of symptoms including pallor, weakness, diaphoresis (sweating), an elevation in respiratory rate and preceded by tachycardia; brady-cardia is common during the act of vomiting.

It is not altogether clear why these symptoms arise during radiotherapy although several theories have been proposed. It is, however, clear that nausea and vomiting occur when the vomiting (emetic) centre is stimulated. This receives afferent stimuli from four main sources: the chemoreceptor trigger zone (CTZ), the vestibular area, the cerebral cortex and peripheral stimuli arising from the gastrointestinal (GI) tract through the vagus nerve. Stimuli transmitted by the vagus reach the brain through the nucleus of the solitary tract (NTS).

The CTZ, located in the area postrema of the IVth ventricle, is stimulated by specific drugs and chemicals and by cellular by-products present in the blood stream. It is believed that cells destroyed by radiation release toxic waste products which stimulate both the CTZ and the vomiting centre (Figure 8.1).

Figure 8.1   Schematic representation of the vomiting reflex

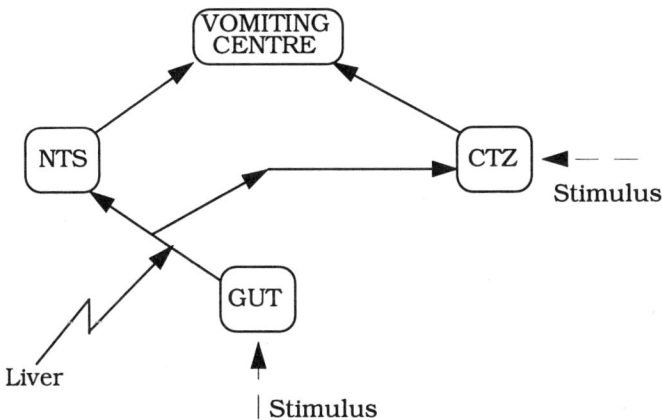

The vomiting centre thus receives stimuli from both the CTZ and NTS; it may also be stimulated by afferent impulses arising in the vestibular area which transmits impulses to both the cerebellum and the emetic centre. This is the basis of motion sickness and may also account for some of the vomiting associated with radiotherapy (Dorr and Fritz, 1980).

The cerebral cortex controls anticipatory and conditioned psychological stimuli and is the mechanism which causes the patient to become nauseated at the sights, sounds and smells associated with the hospital *per se* or the radiotherapy department in particular. Such effects are particularly likely if the patient has previously associated radiation with these symptoms.

The frequency, duration and severity of nausea and vomiting are subject to considerable individual variation and not all patients will be affected. In general, the vomiting associated with radiotherapy is less severe than that caused by cancer chemotherapy although the number of emetic episodes may be greater as a course of radiotherapy can involve 30-40 individual fractionated treatments. Those receiving hyperfractionated therapy (e.g. CHART) may experience greater amounts of nausea and vomiting (Table 8.1).

Table 8.1   Factors potentiating nausea and vomiting in radiotherapy

Site of radiation	e.g. Abdomen and pelvis Para-aortic region Hypochondrium/epigastrium Cranium Wide mediastinal fields
Field size	The greater the volume of tissue irradiated the greater the likelihood of nausea and vomiting.
Dose/fraction	a. The higher the dose the greater the amount of vomiting. b. The greater the number of fractions the greater the likelihood of nausea and vomiting. c. Hyperfractionation potentiates both nausea and vomiting.
Age	Children appear to experience less nausea and vomiting than adults.
Anxiety	Greater levels of anxiety or apprehension lead to greater levels of nausea and vomiting.

Indigestion and nausea are most likely during the first 1-3 weeks of therapy and, once cellular breakdown occurs, may develop as part of the general response to radiotherapy. Whatever their cause, they are extremely disturbing and may necessitate considerable changes in normal patterns of activity. They will interfere with food consumption and, if prolonged, further compromise the patient's nutritional status leading to weight loss and malnutrition. They may lead to dehydration through fluid loss or a failure to maintain fluid intake and, through a loss of gastric secretions, cause fluid and electrolyte imbalance.

Control of nausea and vomiting is, therefore, essential to enhance both physiological and psychological comfort, prevent malnutrition and dehydration, maintain mobility and eliminate fatigue; appropriate care will enable therapy to continue.

Care of the patient suffering nausea and vomiting

The care required includes supportive measures and medication to alleviate the symptoms; nutritional status must be closely monitored (Ch 14). Close observation and assessment may be valuable in preventing both indigestion and nausea which may, for example, be associated with ingestion of certain foods or drugs that may be withheld. Specific factors aggravating nausea and vomiting are:

1. Food and drink.
2. Movement or position change.
3. The mention or sight of chemotherapeutic drugs.
4. Equipment (e.g. syringes or radiotherapy machines).
5. Specific odours.

Measures appropriate in managing indigestion and nausea will vary depending upon the individual concerned. Certain general principles can however, be applied. These include the following:

1. Ensure that patients are aware that these symptoms may arise as a result of treatment and do not, of necessity, indicate further symptoms/spread of the disease. Stress that this is subject to considerable individual variation and that not all patients are affected.
2. Explore remedies that have previously been found helpful in relieving indigestion and/or nausea. Are they appropriate for use in the current situation?
3. Record the onset, duration and intensity of symptoms. Identify any aggravating factors. Evaluate the response to

medical and nursing intervention.

4. Encourage the regular use of prescribed antiemetic therapy. Such drugs appear to work more effectively when taken regularly to maintain optimal blood levels. Ensure that the patient is aware of the possible adverse reactions that may be associated with the antiemetic concerned and is instructed to report any side-effects. Re-evaluate antiemetic therapy regularly.

5. Encourage the patient to rest in a comfortable position, where possible in a quiet and peaceful environment. Ensure that the environment is clean, comfortable and odour-free. Nausea can be triggered by unpleasant sights and smells. Have a vomit bowl nearby but out of sight; some patients may prefer this to be visible and readily available.

6. Provide fresh air by enabling the patient to sit near an open window or even, weather permitting, out of doors.

7. Some patients will find that they are unable to eat for some hours after treatment. Such patients should be encouraged to consume a large and nutritious meal 3-4 hours before radiotherapy and then eat very light meals or snacks every 2-3 hours throughout the day. Liquid nutritional supplements may be valuable (see Ch 14).

8. Encourage experimentation with different foods served at different temperatures until acceptable foods are identified.

9. Use distraction techniques to reduce feelings of nausea. Listening to music, a favourite television programme or talking to nurses, relatives or friends can all provide distraction.

Behavioural techniques, such as hypnosis, guided imagery (visualisation) and progressive muscle relaxation have been used to reduce nausea and control vomiting, particularly with regard to that induced by cancer chemotherapy (Redd and Hendler, 1983). However, their use is controversial and often discouraged, perhaps because they are not really understood. When used by a properly trained and prepared member of the health care team, they are not harmful and may provide the patient with a sense of control over his symptoms. Such techniques are, however, time-demanding and require a one-to-one approach; this may be why they are rarely used within National Health Care provision; they are, however, widely used by many so-called 'alternative' practitioners.

When vomiting is the prevalent symptom additional interventions and observations will be required:

1. The frequency of vomiting, as well as the amount and type of vomit, must be carefully monitored.
2. An accurate fluid balance chart must be maintained and the patient carefully observed for signs of dehydration and electrolyte imbalance (Table 8.2).
3. Encourage the patient to refrain from eating whilst vomiting persists, Advise him to drink as much as possible, sipping liquids slowly.
4. Frequent mouth care and mouthwashes must be offered to maintain comfort particularly after episodes of vomiting.
5. Stay with the patient during episodes of vomiting thus providing both physical and psychological support.

When the condition is severe intravenous fluids may be necessary to replace electrolytes or to prevent or correct dehydration; total parenteral nutrition may be required.

Table 8.2   Signs and symptoms of dehydration (fluid deficit)

Thirst
Poor skin turgor
Dryness of the skin and mucous membranes
Decreased salivation and oral discomfort
Tongue dry and furrowed
Dysphagia, particularly of solid foods
Concentrated urine of a high specific gravity (>1030)
Constipation, production of hard, dry stools; faecal impaction
Eyes appear sunken
Elevated body temperature
Blood pressure and pulse volume normal in early stages
Apprehension and restlessness
Apathy, weakness and disorientation
Late stages
Oliguria - may lead to acidosis
Eyes severely sunken
Blood pressure and pulse rate and volume fall
Coma
Laboratory findings
Elevated haemoglobin
Hypernatraemia
Hypokalaemia

Antiemetic therapy
Since there is considerable individual variation in the incidence and severity of nausea and vomiting it is not possible to suggest any one drug that will be appropriate for all patients. It may, therefore, take several attempts before a suitable and effective drug is identified. On occasions, a combination of drugs, or an antiemetic in conjunction with a sedative or antihistamine, will be required.

Most of the currently available antiemetics are dopamine receptor antagonists (e.g. substituted benzamides, butyrophenones and phenothiazines). As a group these drugs share many common side-effects (Table 8.3) including extra-pyramidal reactions (EPRs) which are most common in children and young adults (Bateman et al, 1989). Examples of possible drugs are discussed below.

Table 8.3   Side-effects of dopamine antagonists

Hypotension
Sedation
Agitation
Extra-pyramidal effects such as: Restlessness
Akasthisia
Oculogyric crises
Torticollis

Metoclopramide is a substituted benzamide with both central and peripheral antiemetic actions. It is a dopamine blocker acting on both the CTZ and the GI tract (Harrington et al, 1983) increasing both gastric emptying and GI motility; at higher doses it is also a 5-HT$_3$ receptor antagonist (see p109). Its side-effects include sedation, diarrhoea and EPRs such as muscle twitching (akasthisia), ataxia and restlessness together with agitation and anxiety. The latter are more common when the drug is given at high doses.

Phenothiazines, such as prochlorperazine, triethylperazine and chlorpromazine, are probably the most widely used antiemetics. They are potent dopamine blockers and are believed to act on the CTZ; they may also have tranquillising effects (e.g. chlorpromazine). These drugs may be administered by a variety of routes and are generally well tolerated. Side-effects are minimal but may include sedation, orthostatic hypotension and occasional EPRs.

Haloperidol is a drug from the butyrophenone group members of which are potent inhibitors of the CTZ through their effects on dopamine receptors. Since they are not associated with hypotension or cardio-respiratory effects, they are useful for elderly or debilitated patients. They may, however, cause insomnia. These drugs are not widely used as antiemetics in the UK.

Antihistamines (e.g. Cyclizine) are effective in decreasing vestibular stimuli. They are poor antiemetics when used alone but may be helpful in increasing the effectiveness of antiemetics and decreasing the incidence of toxic effects. Their action as histamine blockers may also be useful in decreasing GI-vagal stimuli although the mechanism through which this is achieved is not known.

Cannabinoids (delta-9-tetrahydrocannabinol), are derived from marijuana, have been shown to possess antiemetic properties which are equivalent or superior to placebo and the phenothiazines (Orr et al, 1980) particularly against the nausea and vomiting associated with cancer chemotherapy (Sallan et al, 1980). They also possess the ability to produce an elevation of mood, sedation and reduced pain recognition as well as an improvement in appetite all of which may be desirable effects in the cancer patient. However, cannabinoids are also associated with significant toxic effects including hypotension, hallucinations, dysphoria and syncope as well as immunodepression so that they should be used with extreme caution particularly in the elderly or debilitated. The patient must be made aware of the possibility of such side-effects. Their use is controversial and it must be remembered that the use of cannabis (marijuana) *per se* is currently illegal in the UK.

5-HT$_3$ receptor antagonists: Serotonin (5-hydroxytryptamine (5-HT)) is an important neurotransmitter, the highest concentration of which is found in the enterochromaffin cells of the intestinal tract where it plays a major role in the nausea and vomiting induced by radiation (Andrew et al, 1988). It seems likely that this is achieved when radiation causes a release of 5-HT from the gut mucosa. This then activates vagal afferent fibres and initiates vomiting. 5-HT$_3$ receptors are also located centrally where they may also play a role in the vomiting reflex. From this it was deduced that blocking the action of such receptors could effectively prevent vomiting and a range of drugs was developed including Ondansetron and Granisetron.

Chemically, Ondansetron is a carbazole derivative which has been shown to control emesis effectively in 97% of affected patients (Priestman et al, 1990). Granisetron is also effective against the nausea arising from total body irradiation. Both drugs are well tolerated and, as they have no effect on dopamine receptors, EPRs are unlikely. The most common side-effects are constipation and headache.

Steroids: Although the mechanism of action is unknown, cortico-steroids may be used as antiemetic agents. Long-term use, however, is undesirable due to their adverse effects on the immune system and the risk of Cushing-like symptoms.

The most effective glucocorticoid steroid used as an antiemetic is dexamethasone which can control chemotherapy-induced emesis in the majority of patients (e.g. Aapro and Alberti, 1981; Cassileth et al, 1983). Methylprednisolone is also used although it is only moderately effective (Rich et al, 1980; Benrubi et al, 1985).

Interventions related to food and drink

As each patient is an individual acceptable foods and drinks may vary so that an individual approach to care is required. Nonetheless, several general principles may be useful.

1. Since patients are often better able to eat before treatment is delivered they should be encouraged to eat their largest meal at this time. Encourage small but frequent snacks or drinks of a high nutrient density following treatment. Foods having a low nutrient content should be discouraged since these will cause satiety and limit the intake of other, more nutritious, foods.

2. Ensure that antiemetic drugs are given as prescribed so that the antiemetic effect is maximal during and immediately after meals.

3. Avoid fatty, spicy, highly salted or sweet foods as well as those with strong odours. Ensure that food smells do not linger since the odour of hot food may aggravate nausea.

4. Foods that are cold or which are served at room temperature are generally tolerated better than hot foods.

5. Bland foods, such as mashed potatoes, cottage cheese, eggs, may be better tolerated.

6. Eating solid foods alone may be better tolerated than when solids and liquids are combined.

7. Encourage the patient to eat and drink slowly taking small mouthfuls and ensuring that these are well chewed before they are swallowed.

8. A clear liquid diet can be used to minimise nausea although

this should not be adhered to for longer than 2-3 days. Fruit juices, carbonated drinks and clear soups may be tolerated. Some patients find that soda water, or a mixture of soda water and milk, has a settling effect.

9. Stressful stimuli may be reduced by manipulating the external environment to remove the sights, smells and sounds which may contribute to the condition.

When vomiting is severe it may be necessary to withhold oral intake gradually reintroducing solid foods in frequent small meals. In this case, intravenous fluids or total parenteral feeding is essential.

EFFECTS ON THE RESPIRATORY TRACT

The effects of radiation on the normal lung are an important factor in determining tolerance to radiation. This is influenced by the treatment volume and the dose of radiation delivered so that the larger the lung volume involved the greater the risk of radiation pneumonitis.

The initial response results in inflammation of the mucosa lining the alveoli; the alveolar sacs become filled with exudate and diffusion of oxygen and carbon dioxide is inhibited. During the intermediate phase, the alveolar walls are infiltrated by fibroblasts so that, if untreated, fibrosis will occur within 6-12 months; chronic fibrotic changes can permanently damage lung function so that symptoms of respiratory failure may develop. The degree may vary in severity and may affect the patient's ability to function and markedly increase the risk of pulmonary infection.

If radiation exposure includes less than 25% of the lung tissue the patient may be asymptomatic even though the chest X-ray may be abnormal. Alternatively, the initial response may result in mild dyspnoea and a non-productive cough. As exposure increases, and radiation affects more than 25% of the lung tissue, the patient may develop a persistent dry cough accompanied by dyspnoea on exertion, weakness and fatigue and, occasionally, pyrexia. The inflammatory response may be reduced by means of steroid therapy; these may also reduce the degree of damage. Pulmonary infection is treated with appropriate antibiotic therapy.

Respiratory effects usually occur within 1-6 months of therapy and may be exacerbated when the patient has chronic pulmonary disease or respiratory tract infection. Administration of the chemotherapeutic agents actinomycin-D or bleomycin can increase the risk of pulmonary toxicity whether these are given before or after therapy.

Effective care of patients with respiratory problems depends on an understanding of the underlying processes as well as of the complications arising from both the disease *per se* and its treatment. Care focuses largely on symptom relief and on prevention of common respiratory difficulties. Individual assessment of respiratory function is essential in planning appropriate care. This relies on identification of those factors which may impair pulmonary function.

Evaluation of lung function depends on a combination of the medical history, physical examination and laboratory data together with simple observation. The findings may fall into 4 common problem areas:

1. Airway obstruction.
2. Hypoventilation and hypoxia.
3. Inadequate clearance of secretions.
4. Respiratory failure.

Since the severity of the dysfunction determines the supportive measures required, for both the relief of symptoms and the degree of assistance needed to maintain normal daily activity, care must be prescribed on an individual basis particularly when the condition is a chronic one. Certain general principles can, however, be applied.

Common respiratory symptoms

Airway obstruction is characterised by its position along the tracheobronchial tree and whether it is an acute or chronic condition. It may arise in the lumen or the wall of the airway itself or outside the tracheobronchial tree (Table 8.4). In general, the more central the obstruction the greater the disturbance to air flow. Management differs depending on whether it is an acute or chronic condition.

In acute obstruction, care is directed towards removing the obstruction (e.g. tumour removal by surgery, chemotherapy or radiotherapy) or by provision of an artificial airway (e.g. a tracheostomy). Chronic obstruction is managed by teaching the patient to identify those factors impairing ventilatory function and to manage these using measures designed to increase expiratory flow and achieve optimal independence with regard to his normal activities of daily living.

Bronchospasm may be treated using drug therapy to promote relaxation of the bronchial muscles and increase vital capacity. Together with breathing exercises and relaxation techniques this will

Table 8.4 **Examples of airway obstruction**

Site of obstruction	Possible causes
Intraluminal	Secretions (mucus plugs)
	Neoplasm
	Foreign bodies
	Pneumonia
Wall of airway	Tumours
	Diffuse disease (e.g. fibrosis, asthma, chronic obstructive airways disease)
Outside tracheobronchial tree	Tumours (e.g. head and neck, thorax, abdomen)

help to decrease anxiety and increase respiratory flow. Airway obstruction will, however, contribute to the development of both hypoventilation and hypoxia since gaseous exchange is inhibited when air movement is decreased. Hypoventilation arises when pulmonary function is such that it is unable to maintain alveolar ventilation at a level appropriate to meet the metabolic demand may be of functional or structural origin.

Functional causes include malnutrition and fatigue. Structural causes include tumours which obstruct the airway and treatment-induced effects, such as pneumonitis and pulmonary fibrosis, which restrict lung expansion and ventilation, or pneumonia when exudate accumulates in the alveoli. Hypoventilation may, in turn, lead to hypoxia, hypercapnia and pneumonia.

A decrease in oxygen tension (hypoxia) can, however, occur even in the absence of hyperventilation due to changes in the cardiovascular-respiratory-haemopoietic system essential to satisfactory tissue oxygenation and appropriate gaseous exchange. As a result, hypoxia may be the result of a variety of causes including:

- Disturbances of the alveolar-capillary membrane, such as those accompanying pulmonary fibrosis or emphysema, when fibrotic changes or oedema of the alveolar walls result in a decrease in the amount of oxygen diffusing into the circulation
- A reduction in cardiac output
- Alterations in blood composition due to anaemia and a subsequent decrease in haemoglobin content. A reduction in the number of erythrocytes, or a less than normal complement of haemoglobin, will reduce the amount of

oxygen that can be taken up by the blood.

Hypoventilation may also lead to hypercapnia, the retention of carbon dioxide (CO_2) in excess of the normal range. Since carbon dioxide is more soluble than oxygen, and diffuses more readily, hypercapnia develops more slowly than hypoxia.

Prevention of hypoventilation, hypoxia and hypercapnia is essential. Symptomatic treatment includes drainage of pleural effusions - which will inhibit thoracic expansion, and use of broncho-dilators, such as orciprenaline or salbutamol, or drugs, such as digoxin, to improve cardiac output. When required, blood trans-fusions can be given to correct anaemia.

Both obstruction of the airway and hypoventilation will inhibit the clearance of secretions from the respiratory tract. Unless preventive measures are taken secretions will accumulate predisposing to the development of pneumonia. When this is combined with immuno-suppression the risk is further increased.

Care is, therefore, directed towards preventing pneumonia and may include the prophylatic use of antibiotics, treatment of the airway obstruction, endotracheal intubation, insertion of a tracheostomy tube to aid the removal of secretions or bronchoscopy designed to remove mucus plugs.

Respiratory failure

Respiratory failure results when the respiratory system is unable to maintain adequate oxygenation and elimination of carbon dioxide. The already compromised patient is at particular risk of respiratory suppression following administration of certain drugs (e.g. narcotics, and some tranquillisers) so that these should be used with caution in affected patients.

Other causes include sepsis within the respiratory tract and interstitial fibrosis, both of which restrict lung expansion, and obstruction of the major airways. Clearly diagnosis and treatment are essential in the care of affected patients. Although detailed discussion of the necessary care and management is outside the scope of this book an outline of the care required is shown in Table 8.5.

Care of the patient with a respiratory disturbance

Improving the quality of life for affected patients is a major aim of care since respiratory disturbances can significantly affect the normal

Table 8.5   Care of patients with respiratory failure

Prevention of infection	Prevent pneumonia as described. Ensure secretions are removed by means of physiotherapy and postural drainage. Use aseptic techniques when suctioning is required.
Positioning **Acute (short-term)**	Turn head laterally with neck extended; inspect mouth for cause of obstruction. Insert artificial airway to relieve obstruction and maintain airway.
Chronic (long-term)	Get patient out of bed to maximise thoracic expansion and improve oxygenation. This will also facilitate removal of secretions. Educate the patient and his family about management and appropriate care.
Oxygenation and mechanical ventilation	Maintain patency of the airway and humidify inhaled air. When mechanical ventilation is employed, ensure endotracheal or tracheostomy tube is well secured. Change ventilator tubing every 24hrs. Improve oxygen-carrying capacity by maintaining haemoglobin within normal limits, improving cardiac output and decreasing the work of breathing.
Prevention of the complications of mechanical ventilation	Maintain patency of the airway and humidify inhaled air. Remove accumulated secretions. Prevent laryngeal or tracheal complications by securing the endotracheal tube, using low pressure cuffs or using minimal pressure occluding volume in the inflating cuff. Prevent barotrauma by minimising peak airway pressure, use of intermittent ventilation, prolonged expiratory time or decreased respiratory rate. Provide for mechanical emergencies - have Ambu-bag and mask at bed side.
Fluid balance	Ensure adequate hydration but restrict fluids if water retention is present. Administer diuretics when prescribed. Minimise the effects of positive pressure breathing; use intermittent mechanical ventilation. Minimise peak airway pressure.
General care	Control pain and stress. Sedate the patient when necessary. Maintain oral hygiene and pressure area care. Provide comfort and reassurance.

pattern of activity and make 'normal' living impossible for the sufferer. The goals of care are, therefore, directed towards this aim and include:

- Promotion of optimal ventilation and oxygenation
- A decrease in the 'work' involved in respiration
- Prevention of infection.

General principles can be applied as well as specific measures designed to overcome particular problems all of which are dependent on as an individual assessment of respiratory function.

Table 8.6 gives an outline of the clinical findings associated with each of the respiratory problems highlighted in the preceding discussion. These will provide a baseline against which to judge future changes, Continued regular assessment will enable evaluation of respiratory function and ensure that changes are identified and, where appropriate, treated at an early stage.

The following parameters will help to detect changes in the respiratory tract and may indicate the presence of pneumonitis:
- Percussion - to identify areas of dullness
- Auscultation - to identify the presence of rhonci and râles
- Observation - to identify changes in the type, frequency and severity of coughing
- X-ray - to identify the presence and/or extent of pneumonitis, fibrosis, infection or obstruction
- Monitoring of blood gases and pH (see Table 8.7).

Pneumonitis may be accompanied by a dry, persistent cough, dyspnoea on exertion, weakness and fatigue and, on occasions, pyrexia. Care is directed towards relief of symptoms as well as an improvement in pulmonary ventilation.

A persistent cough is both debilitating and disabling and can, in itself, promote fatigue and exhaustion. Its relief is, therefore, a major aim. Humidifying the air the patient breathes can play a major role in decreasing the frequency of the cough. Inspired air is usually moistened within the respiratory tract by the moisture evaporated from the mucosal surfaces. Inflammation results in water depletion so that the mucus becomes viscous and impairs ciliary activity. The retention of this tenacious mucus increases airway resistance and promotes infection.

Humidification is, therefore, an important part of care. Various methods can be used for humidification. The choice depends mainly on:
- Whether or not the upper airway is bypassed
- The degree of mucosal dehydration.

Table 8.6   Assessment of pulmonary function: clinical signs

	Medical history	Physical examination	Arterial blood gases	Chest X-ray	Pulmonary function tests
Airway obstruction	Dyspnoea and/or shortness of breath, cough haemoptysis, and recurrent upper respiratory tract infections	Cyanosis, increased rate of respiration, prolonged expiration. Use of accessory muscles of respiration. Stridor, tracheal shift. Flat or hyperresonant percussion; rhonci, râles and wheezing. Signs of consolidation, marked respiratory effort without air movement.	Po_2 - decreased Pco_2 - may be increased or decreased.	May show tumour, pneumonia or chronic obstructive airways disease.	Indicative of an obstructive defect.
Hypoxia and hypo-ventilation	Dyspnoea, tachypnoea, headache, lethargy, fatigue and restlessness, irritability and confusion.	Coma, cyanosis, tachy-cardia. Hypertension followed by hypo-tension. Decreased respiratory expansion, decreased breath sounds. Reduced diaphragmatic movement. Rhonci, râles, wheezing and signs of consolidation	Po_2 - decreased Pco_2 - may be increased	May show pulmonary oedema or fibrosis, tumour or pneumonia.	Indicative of an obstructive or restrictive defect.
Inadequate clearance of secretions	Cough with/without sputum. Change in colour, odour or consistency of sputum. Pyrexia. History of smoking and/or chronic obstructive airways disease.	Cyanosis. Increased work of breathing and increased respiratory rate. Use of accessory muscles of respiration Rhonci, râles, wheezing and signs of consolidation; systemic signs of dehydration.			
Respiratory failure	Rapid and progressive air hunger. Restlessness and confusion. Profuse sweating, headache. May also have a history of any of the symptoms listed above.	Tachycardia, hypotension, cyanosis Confusion, tremors. Decreased respiratory effort and respiratory rate. Papilloedema.	Po_2 - decreased Pco_2 - may be increased or decreased.	May show tumour, fibrosis, pneumonia or oedema.	Indicative of an obstructive or restrictive defect.

Table 8.7   Interrelationships between Po_2, Pco_2, pH and respiration

	Effects of decrease	Effect of increase
Po_2	Stimulates respiration; CO_2 'blown off'	Increase has little effect on respiration
Pco_2	Inhibition of respiration. When Pco_2 = 30mmHg or less ventilation decreases to 25% of normal	Stimulates respiration. When Pco_2 reaches 50mmHg, ventilatory rate will triple
pH	Respiration stimulated when pH is below 7.41; if pH <7.20 pulmonary ventilation will quadruple.	When pH >7.41 respiration is inhibited. If pH >7.50 pulmonary ventilation decreased by 50%

When oxygen is required, bubbling it through water will increase its vapour content; the amount of water absorbed can be increased by heating the water. A more efficient method is delivery of water in an aerosol or nebulised form when the nebuliser produces a coarse spray of fluid that is directed into a stream of rapidly moving gas which is, subsequently, directed onto the walls of the container to reduce the size of the water particles. The usual diluent is sterile water although normal saline may be used. Hypertonic saline will promote liquefaction and elimination of accumulated secretions; this should not, however, be used unless prescribed by the physician.

Medications, such as bronchodilators [e.g. salbutamol], may also be given in nebulised form thus avoiding systemic administration and the associated side-effects. A high fluid intake (3000ml/day) will, in conjunction with high humidity, help to liquefy secretions so that, unless such a fluid intake is contraindicated, at least 1000ml should be taken in each eight hour period. Warm fluids will be soothing when the cough is particularly persistent. Alternatively, when the cough is inhibiting normal rest and sleep, a cough suppressant (such as codeine linctus) may be given; cough lozenges or boiled sweets may also be helpful. Clearly any irritant substances in the environment (e.g. cigarette smoke or strong perfume) should be avoided.

The patient should be encouraged to adopt a position that promotes optimal thoracic expansion and, therefore, improves both oxygenation and removal of any accumulated secretions. Ideally he will sit out of bed with his head and back bent slightly forward, his arms relaxed and supported (e.g. leaning on the forearm or elbow) and his feet flat on a firm surface. A similar posture can be adopted in bed. In general, the patient will be the best guide as to what position is the most comfortable; this will probably be that which provides the best alveolar ventilation. Successful relief of coughing will help to promote rest and sleep and to reduce fatigue.

Prevention of infection

All the respiratory problems discussed carry with them a significant risk of pneumonia; prevention of infection is, therefore, an essential part of care. It is essential that strict asepsis is maintained when caring for patients with respiratory disturbances both to decrease exposure to potentially infective organisms and to prevent cross-infection. This is particularly important when the patient has a temporary or permanent tracheostomy or is also suffering from bone marrow depression or is otherwise immunosuppressed. On occasions, protective isolation (reverse barrier care) will be required. Where possible, however, the length of the hospital stay should be reduced.

Immunocompetence should be enhanced by ensuring that optimal nutritional status is maintained (see Ch 14) and that the patient has adequate rest and sleep. The individual must be advised to avoid contact with any person (hospital staff, relatives or friends) thought to be suffering a respiratory tract infection, influenza or a cold.

Since the patient's respiration is often shallow, due to weakness and pain, ensure that secretions do not accumulate. The patient should be encouraged to take regular deep breaths inhaling deeply and relaxing the abdominal muscles. He should then lean forward and exhale as much as possible through pursed lips. Exhalation is more effective when the abdominal muscles are contracted so that pressure exerted on the lower abdomen will promote compression and aid in the elevation of the diaphragm during exhalation.

Breathing exercises should be carried out 2 or 3 times daily; their effectiveness may be increased if they are preceded by administration of a prescribed bronchodilator via a nebuliser.

Coughing is essential for removal of secretions from the respiratory tract and should not be suppressed unless it is non-productive or excessive and exhausting. The patient should be taught to cough effectively. Where possible the patient should be in the sitting position and deep inspiration should be followed by a series of small, short coughs (short coughs require less energy and are less likely to cause airway collapse than a single, large and forceful exhalation). Coughing can be assisted manually in patients with weak abdominal muscles. The patient must be closely observed for signs of fatigue

119

and allowed to rest when necessary; pain or unusual fatigue when coughing must be reported to the physician. The physiotherapist will advise when specific care and/or postural drainage is required.

Coughing can be stimulated by irritation of the pharynx using, for example, the tip of a suction catheter or application of digital pressure over the trachea just above the medial clavicular prominence. Prolonging exhalation may also stimulate coughing since the increased flow of air may act to dry and irritate the mucosa. When these measures are unsuccessful deep suctioning will be required.

Alternatively, when efficient access to the retained pulmonary secretions is essential to prevent the development of more serious respiratory problems (e.g. pneumonia), a tracheostomy may be performed. A tracheostomy may also be needed when the upper airway is obstructed by a tumour or laryngeal oedema at least until treatment effectively eliminates or reduces the size of the obstruction.

References

Aapro MS, Alberti DS, 1981, High-dose dexamethasone for prevention of cis-platin-induced vomiting, Cancer Chemotherapeutic Pharmacology, **7**, 11-14.

Andrew PLR, Rapeport WG, Sanger GJ, 1988, Neuropharmacology of emesis induced by anti-cancer therapy, Trends in Pharmaceutical Science, **9**, 334-341.

Bateman DN, Darling WM, Boys R, Rawlins MD, 1989, Extra-pyramidal reactions to metoclopramide and prochlorperazine, Quarterly Journal of Medicine, **264**, 307-311.

Benrubi GI, Norwell M, Nuss RC, Robinson H, 1985, The use of methylprednisolone and metoclopramide in control of emesis in patients receiving cis-platinum, Gynecologic Oncology, **21**, 306-313.

Cassileth A, Lusk EJ, Torri S et al, 1983, Antiemetic efficacy of dexamethasone therapy in patients receiving cancer chemotherapy, Archives of Internal Medicine, **143**, 1347-1359.

Dorr R, Fritz W, 1980, Cancer Chemotherapy Handbook, Elsevier North Holland Inc., New York.

Finkelstein E, 1986, Nifedipine for radiation and oesophagitis, Lancet, i, 1205-1206 (Letter to the Editor).

Harrington RA, Hamilton CW, Brogden RN et al, 1983,

Metoclopramide: an updated review of its pharmacological properties and clinical use Drugs, **25**, 451-494.

Orr LE, Mckerman JF, Blonne B, 1980, Antiemetic effect of tetra-hydrocannabinol, Archives of Internal Medicine, **140**, 1431-1433.

Priestman TJ, Roberts JT, Lucraft H et al, 1990, Results of a randomized, double-blind comparative study of Ondansetron and metoclopramide in the prevention of nausea and vomiting following high-dose upper abdominal irradiation, Clinical Oncology, **2**, 71-75.

Redd WH, Hendler CS, 1983, Behavioural medicine in comprehensive cancer treatment, Journal of Psychosocial Oncology, **1**, 3-17.

Rich WM, Abdulhayoglu G, DiSaia PJ, 1980, Methylprednisolone as an antiemetic during cancer chemotherapy - a pilot study, Gynecologic Oncology, **9**, 193-198.

Sallan SE, Cronin C, Zelen M, Zinberg NE, 1980, Antiemetics in patients receiving chemotherapy for cancer, New England Journal of Medicine, **302**, 135-138.

Stevens KR, 1989, The oesophagus. In: Moss WT, Cox JD (Editors), Radiation Oncology, Rationale, Techniques, Results (Sixth edition), CV Mosby, St Louis.

Strohl R, 1988, The nursing role in radiation oncology. Symptom management of acute and chronic reactions, Oncology Nursing Forum, **15**, 429-434.

Unsawasdi T, Valdivieso M, Barkley HT, 1985, Esophageal complications from combined chemoradiotherapy (cyclophosphamide + adriamycin + cisplatin + XRT) in the treatment of non-small cell lung cancer, International Journal of Radiation Oncology, Biology and Physics, **11**, 511-519.

CHAPTER 9   RADIATION TO THE ABDOMEN AND PELVIS

Since the intestinal mucosa is second only to the bone marrow in its sensitivity to radiation, curative doses of irradiation, particularly when directed at any portion of the gastrointestinal tract can have marked toxic effects many of which prove to be a limiting factor to intensive treatment. Acute or chronic damage may follow radiation to the abdomen and pelvis arising during, immediately or many years after treatment. The extent of the damage is dependent on the dose, time and fractionation of the administered dose as well as the area of the treatment field.

EFFECTS OF RADIATION ON THE STOMACH

Radiation-induced damage to the stomach appears to be dose-dependent and results in histological changes which primarily affect glandular tissue. All gastric secretions including mucus, pepsin and free hydrochloric acid are reduced following a dose of about 1600cGy delivered in approximately 10 days. This may be accompanied by an asymptomatic gastritis, due to mucositis, or result in oedema, hyper-aemia, microscopic haemorrhages and exudate which can cause nausea, dyspepsia and, on occasions, pyloric spasm; antiemetics may be required. Severe anorexia and an associated weight loss may follow; the care described for the anorexic individual (Ch 6) is appropriate when caring for affected patients.

High doses of irradiation may result in ulceration manifested by severe, unremitting epigastric pain, bleeding and haematemesis, and progressive weight loss. Since such ulcers often fail to respond to conventional therapy partial or total gastrectomy may be necessary. A bland diet and regular antacid administration are appropriate preventive measures.

EFFECTS ON THE LIVER

Although the liver is a moderately radiosensitive organ, the main effects of radiation are due to vascular injury (Hilderley, 1992). Rarely, radiation at doses in excess of 2500cGy will cause hepatitis. Hepatitis is characterised by abdominal pain and jaundice and accompanied by hepatomegaly, ascites and a concurrent weight gain. Late effects include fibrosis, and cirrhosis; portal hypertension may follow severe fibrosis (D'Angio and Pearson, 1975)

EFFECTS OF RADIATION ON THE SMALL INTESTINE

Since the small intestinal mucosa is second only to the bone marrow in its sensitivity to radiation, curative doses of irradiation may cause significant damage, particularly when this is directed at any portion of the GI tract. Since even a small treatment field is likely to include a large area of the intestinal mucosa, this may prove to be a limiting factor to intensive treatment (Holmes and Dickerson, 1988). Radiation-induced damage arises primarily from effects on normal tissues; its extent is dependant on the dose, time and fractionation of the administered dose as well as the volume of the treatment field. Acute or chronic effects may arise during, immediately following or many years after radiotherapy.

The cells of the intestinal mucosa are highly proliferative and rapidly dividing, being replaced about every 2 days; mucosal damage can occur rapidly after even low doses of radiation. This results in inflammatory lesions, delayed or arrested mitosis and submucosal oedema. Initially, this causes retention of the intestinal content by reducing propulsive mobility. The gut later becomes dilated and flaccid and diarrhoea becomes the prominent symptom.

Irradiation involving the connective tissue provokes an initial inflammation which later leads to thickening of the collagen and other elastic fibres so that clinically detectable fibrosis is common, particularly after large doses (>5000cGy) (Ruccione and Weinberg, 1989). These effects may persist and progress long after treatment has ceased and may not be detectable until some years later. Tissues affected by such damage are fibrotic and poorly vascularised; this may form the basis of many of the late complications of therapy such as necrosis, fibrosis and stenosis. In addition, such tissues are less resistant to mechanical injury and infection so that, following radio-therapy, even minor trauma or infection may induce serious complications in an already compromised tissue.

As a result, patients undergoing abdominal or pelvic irradiation often experience nausea and vomiting, severe diarrhoea, abdominal distension, cramps and flatulence. The time of onset and duration diarrhoea are variable; it may clear spontaneously after 4-5 days or persist long after treatment has been completed and be unresponsive to conventional therapies (Mennie et al, 1975). Radiation enteritis may, occasionally present as partial or total intestinal obstruction.

Given the severity of radiation-induced damage to the intestinal mucosa it is not surprising that malabsorption is another common side-effect when significant amounts of the small intestine are included in the treatment field. This is due not only to diarrhoea, but also to direct effects on the absorptive surface of the intestinal mucosa the structure of which is designed to enhance absorption through its large surface area. The villi and microvilli are responsible for both digestion and absorption of food since the microvilli produce many of the enzymes necessary for digestion before nutrients are absorbed by the villi. The epithelial cells of the villi divide rapidly to replace those cells lost as part of the normal sloughing process; they are, therefore, particularly vulnerable to the effects of radiation.

Thus, when an area of the mucosa is exposed to radiation, the villi rapidly become flattened and atrophic, the mucosa becomes ulcerated and the absorptive surface is reduced. At the same time, the composition and concentration of enzymes in the mucosal cells is reduced (e.g. Jervis et al, 1977). As a result, neither food nor water can be adequately digested nor absorbed exacerbating the diarrhoea and compromising nutritional status.

Malnutrition is a recognised hazard of abdo-pelvic radiotherapy, particularly in those receiving doses of radiation in the region of 5000-6000cGy (see Ch 14). However, most patients receiving such therapy will experience no more than a small degree of diarrhoea and abdominal cramping; some may develop nausea and/or anorexia. A small, but nevertheless significant, number may develop severe symptoms.

EFFECTS OF RADIATION ON THE LARGE INTESTINE
Little digestion or absorption take place in the large intestine although it acts as a 'reservoir' for the faecal mass from which both water and electrolytes are absorbed. Irradiation may disrupt the mucosa leading to inadequate absorption so that diarrhoea results.

Clearly, symptoms such as diarrhoea may be disabling and debilitating and may result in malnutrition as the patient ingests less food and is less able to digest and absorb those nutrients available. This may be so severe as to contribute to an early death in affected patients although this may also be due to diarrhoea which can result in terminal losses of electrolytes and water. Yet, to some extent, such effects are to be expected if an adequate dose of radiation is to be administered to a tumour lying in or near the alimentary tract.

Recognition of the risk of malnutrition, effective monitoring and the instigation of appropriate preventive measures and/or nutritional support, therefore, form an essential part of care (see Ch 14).

Care of the patient with diarrhoea

Since diarrhoea is a symptom that can be anticipated in those undergoing abdo-pelvic irradiation, particularly when doses in the region of 2500cGy are to be employed, the patient must be informed of the likelihood of its occurrence so that it is not seen as an exacerbation of his disease. This may cause an increase in the usual number of bowel movements or result in the passage of a large amount of loose, watery stools accompanied by intestinal cramping. Occasionally, treatment must be halted to allow the gut to recover from radiation-induced damage. Diarrhoea is a debilitating and distressing side-effect that may significantly alter the patient's pattern of activity so that comprehensive supportive care may be needed.

A thorough assessment must be carried out before the start of treatment to provide a baseline against which to judge the extent and severity of diarrhoea. This should be designed to establish the usual pattern of elimination, the current nutritional status and the patient's usual coping strategies so that he can, when necessary, be helped to come to terms with his symptoms.

The patient should be instructed to keep a record of the frequency and characteristics of any diarrhoea and to report its occurrence to a member of the caring team; stools should also be observed for the presence of blood. Appropriate antidiarrhoeal medication (e.g. loperamide hydrochloride) can help to reduce diarrhoea and may also help to relieve abdominal cramping. Various drugs (e.g. aspirin) may be used to reduce inflammation. Drug effectiveness must be monitored and adjustments made to the therapeutic regime as required.

When diarrhoea is severe or intractable, physical care must be directed towards reducing the activity of the bowel. Bed rest will be necessary although this may be difficult to achieve in the patient with diarrhoea; hospitalisation may be required. Bed rest in the debilitated patient carries the risk of pressure sores so that pressure area care is essential particularly with regard to the anal area which may be inflamed, sore and excoriated from diarrhoea and accidental leakage.

Radiation to the abdomen and pelvis

Loss of bowel control may be very embarrassing and stressful for the patient who may, for example, require a bedpan at meal times when other patients are eating and when he may be concerned about his 'antisocial behaviour'. Distress may be increased if a bedpan is not available and soiling of the bed results. This may be interpreted as a return to childhood and lead to feelings of low self-esteem so that the patient may require considerable emotional support and reassurance. Sensitive care can help to reduce these concerns. For example, the nurse's attitude is particularly important since the patient will require reassurance that giving and clearing bedpans and changing beds are something which nurses expect to do rather than an unpleasant chore. A clean, covered bedpan or commode can be left at the bed side to reassure the patient. An air freshener should be available.

Large amounts of fluid may be lost causing dehydration and electrolyte imbalance so that accurate records of fluid balance must be maintained and the patient closely observed for signs of toxicity and dehydration (see Table 8.2). The patient should be encouraged to drink a minimum of 3000ml each day and must be advised not to restrict this to water but to consume other liquids, such as fruit juices, clear soups and bouillon to increase the sodium and potassium intake. Carbonated drinks should not be encouraged, unless they are allowed to 'go flat' since they may exacerbate diarrhoea. Fluids should be served at room temperature since extremes of temperature may also aggravate diarrhoea.

Electrolyte balance must be closely monitored and losses, especially of potassium and sodium, should be replaced early. Initially this can be achieved by including foods high in potassium in the diet (e.g. baked potatoes, bananas, orange juice) or by additional potassium supplements. Where necessary intravenous fluid replacement should be given using saline solutions with added potassium. If intravenous feeding must be continued for longer than 72 hours, 3% amino acid solutions may be given to prevent protein catabolism particularly when food intake is restricted as, for some patients, complete bowel rest may be required. In this case, total parenteral nutrition, as described in Ch 14, may be necessary. For others, a liquid diet may be beneficial and use of low osmolality, low residue nutritional formulae may help maintain the nutrient intake but, again, total parenteral nutrition may be required when malabsorption is present and weight loss continues.

When an oral diet can be tolerated the diet generally adopted is one that will leave very little residue in the intestinal tract and which is high in protein and carbohydrate. Foods that are either irritant or stimulating to the GI tract should be avoided and soft, bland, easily digestible foods selected.

The diet outlined in Table 9.1 is appropriate although, for some patients, milk and milk products should be avoided since they may exacerbate diarrhoea. This is due to the effects of radiation on the GI mucosa which cause changes in the concentration of the digestive enzymes and an absence of lactase, the enzyme necessary for digestion of milk. Lactose intolerance means that undigested lactose will ferment in the intestine causing distension, flatulence and severe cramping. Affected patients may, however, be able to tolerate yoghurt and other fermented milk products since lactose may be destroyed by the action of lactobacilli, the microorganism used to promote fermentation. Milk substitutes and non-dairy creamers can be used to make food and drinks more palatable. When required, low osmolality, lactose-free nutritional supplements can be given. In general, individual patients will be the best guide as to which foods are acceptable and do not exacerbate the symptoms.

Diarrhoea, and the concurrent debilitation, are exhausting and fatigue is a common sequelae. Frequent rest periods must be planned. Mucosal irritation must be carefully assessed and perianal care must be meticulous to prevent the occurrence of secondary, opportunistic infection. This will also aid patient comfort and help to prevent the development of pressure sores.

CHRONIC RADIATION ENTERITIS

When the symptoms persist, chronic radiation enteritis may be diagnosed. This results in severe weight loss and debilitation together with megaloblastic anaemia. Radiation-induced damage may also lead to stricture, ulceration, the development of fistulae and intestinal obstruction. Nutritional rehabilitation and surgical intervention are, therefore, important aspects of the care of the affected patient.

EFFECTS ON THE URINARY TRACT

Since the epithelial cells lining the bladder are rapidly dividing they are particularly sensitive to irradiation so that its acute effects may result in cystitis and urethritis. Such effects are infrequent but distressing. Inflammation is generally confined to the mucosa and

Table 9.1   **Diet suitable for the patient with severe diarrhoea**

	Permitted	Not allowed
Meat, poultry, fish, eggs, meat substitutes	Any meat, poultry or fish, eggs, cottage cheese, hard cheese	Fried meats or sausages. Dried peas, beans and legumes. Nuts and seeds
Dairy products - milk, cheese, yoghurt	Cottage cheese, hard cheese, yoghurt - without fruit.	Yoghurt with fruit
Breads and cereals	White bread or rolls, cream crackers, rusks, water biscuits, plain biscuits, rice, pasta, corn, well-cooked oatmeal	Wholegrain cereals and bread, whole-meal pasta, cereals with dried fruit and/or nuts.
Vegetables	Potatoes without skin, asparagus, squash or marrow, green beans, carrots.	Other vegetables, dried beans, peas, nuts, seeds, peanut butter (crunchy) and
Fruit	Bananas, apple sauce, apples (in any form, cooked or raw), grape juice and other fruit juice (strained). Avocados.	All other fruit.
Desserts	Any desserts without fruit, seeds or nuts (e.g. milk puddings, egg custards, ice creams, sponge puddings).	Fruit, nuts and seeds other than those identified.
Soups	Creamed or clear soups not based on vegetables	Vegetable soups except those made with permitted vegetables.
Snacks	Plain biscuits, potato crisps, pretzels and rice snacks.	Nuts and seeds. Popcorn.
Drinks	Any drinks other than those listed in the next column.	Coffee, hot chocolate, beer, liquor, carbonated drinks.

Add flavourings and seasoning to taste; avoid pickles, relishes, gravy with vegetables or made from vegetable stock. Omit jams with seeds, popcorn and coconut.

submucosa which become hyperaemic and oedematous. Scattered haemorrhagic areas may be present and sloughing of the epithelium may lead to the development of small ulcerative lesions. If the condition persists the inflammation may extend into the bladder musculature causing fibrosis which will reduce the bladder capacity increasing the problems of frequency and may necessitate permanent catheterisation.

Cystitis is characterised by frequency of micturition and an urgency to void (which may be almost continuous), dysuria and, at times, particularly when an infection is present, pus, bacteria and mucus will be found in the urine. Micturition may cause burning, acute discomfort and pain and low back pain may be present; haematuria is not uncommon. Passing urine is usually easy and pain-free and often provides a sense of relief. Individuals vary in the number of times urinate each day establishing a personal pattern. Most people void on waking and before retiring at night and, usually, several times during the day depending on both the fluid intake and on personal habit. The 'average' person passes urine once every 3-4 hours during the day and rarely at night unless a large quantity of fluid is consumed.

Changes in urinary function may lead to feelings of shame, particularly if the symptoms lead to incontinence; embarrassment and depression are common sequelae and the symptoms themselves can lead to marked changes in the normal pattern of activity. As a result, the patient may require considerable emotional support. Such symptoms are extremely disturbing and distressing for the patient and must be recognised as such.

Care of the patient with cystitis

When the patient has urinary dysfunction a careful assessment is indicated to enable an appropriate care plan to be designed to minimise discomfort, promote continence and aid both psychological and physical comfort. The patient must also be assured that this is a side-effect of his treatment and does not, of necessity, indicate disease progression. He must, therefore, be 'forewarned' of the possibility that cystitis may occur and be taught appropriate self-care measures to help to reduce its impact. To rule out infection, a mid-stream specimen of urine should be obtained for culture and sensitivity; where appropriate, antibiotic therapy should be given. More commonly no infection is found. Treatment is symptomatic comprising antispasmodic agents and urinary antiseptics.

A high fluid intake should be encouraged; an intake of 1000ml every eight hours (3000ml/day) is an effective regimen. This keeps the urine osmolality low, facilitates urination and helps to reduce the risk of urinary tract infection. The patient may also find it helpful to avoid substances known to be irritant to the bladder mucosa (e.g. tea, coffee, all alcoholic drinks, spicy foods and tobacco).

The risk of infection can also be reduced by teaching the patient measures designed to maintain an acidic urine (pH <7) as this will inhibit the rate of bacterial replication in the bladder. Some workers suggest this is best achieved by giving daily doses of ascorbic acid (vitamin C) although the evidence regarding its efficacy is somewhat equivocal. It is believed that dietary measures may be effective in acidifying the urine so that the nurse or dietician can help the patient to select an appropriate diet. Daily measurement of the urinary pH will indicate whether these measures are effective.

Acid-base balance in foods. The potential acidity or alkalinity of a food refers to the metabolic end-products of that food after digestion, absorption and utilisation. Most fruits and vegetables are rich in potassium, calcium and magnesium and produce acids that can be used by the body (e.g. carbonic acid). The end-products requiring excretion are, therefore, of an alkaline nature and so will decrease the acidity of the urine. As a result, most fruits and vegetables should be restricted when an acid urine is required the exceptions being corn, plums, prunes and cranberries. A diet providing large quantities of protein will, however, yield acidic waste products due to their high phosphorus, sulphur and iron content. Appropriate foods include eggs, meat, fish, poultry, milk and milk products, cereal and cereal products, and bread. Neutral foods (i.e. which produce neither an excess of alkaline nor acid residue) include sugar, tapioca, tea and coffee, butter and cooking oils, lard, cornflour and plain boiled sweets. This means that the required high energy, high protein diet, necessary for both cellular repair and regeneration and to maintain an optimal nutritional status, can be achieved despite the need for some dietary restrictions to alleviate the symptoms of cystitis.

Many texts refer to the value of cranberry juice as a urinary acidulant as this contains quinic acid, which is metabolised to form hippuric acid and excreted in the urine. However, Sobota (1984) has indicated that it has only a small effect on urinary pH. It seems clear that cranberry juice does, indeed, inhibit bacterial growth and adherence to the bladder mucosa (Zafriri, 1989; Nazarko, 1995) and so may be useful in treating cystitis due to bacterial agents; its value in radiation-induced cystitis has yet to be demonstrated.

Pain may be significant so that analgesics may be required. Relief may also be achieved by sitting in a warm bath. Good personal hygiene and efficient cleansing of the perineum, especially after defaecation, are, however, extremely important in preventing ascending infection. Satisfactory cleansing is often difficult for the ill patient or for the weak or handicapped so that it then becomes the nurses' responsibility to see that the patient is thoroughly cleansed.

Catheterisation. Wherever possible the use of indwelling catheters should be avoided since their use is associated with bacteriuria, febrile urinary tract infection and sepsis. For the male, condom catheter drainage may be effective and, in the female, appropriate padding and incontinence devices may prove acceptable alternatives. However, there will be occasions when catheterisation is necessary and when specific care will be required. Great care should be taken to prevent trauma during both catheter placement and throughout the period during which the catheter remains in place (Table 9.2). The patient must be closely observed for signs of retention following removal of the catheter.

Table 9.2   Care of the patient with an indwelling catheter

a. During placement:	Use strict asepsis Use generous amounts of sterile lubricant Use the smallest possible catheter Do not force the catheter
b. Subsequent care:	**Males:** Secure catheter to abdomen to prevent rubbing of the penis at the scrotal junction. **Females:** Secure catheter to thigh to avoid pulling.
c. Prevention of Infection:	Keep the drainage system closed at all times. Obtain specimens through the needle aspiration port. Ensure drainage bag is below the level of the bladder at all times. Maintain accurate records of fluid intake and output and ensure an adequate fluid intake. Ensure both the catheter and meatus are kept clean at all times Ensure urine is kept acid Remove catheter as soon as possible.

RADIATION NEPHRITIS

Radiation nephritis may arise (Ruccione and Weinberg, 1989) particularly when the dose delivered exceeds 2000cGy; the risk is increased by administration of radiation-enhancing chemotherapy (Moore and Ruccione, 1992) and by doses >5000cGy (Ruccione and Weinberg, 1989). Nephritis is characterised by proteinuria, hypertension that can usually be controlled with antihypertensive drugs, and anaemia.

Renal function must be carefully monitored and appropriate treatment instigated. Rarely, chronic nephritis may occur leading to renal failure and cardiovascular damage.

EFFECTS ON BONE AND CARTILAGE

The major effects of irradiation on bone and cartilage are those affecting children, although the use of megavoltage techniques and protracted treatment schedules has considerably reduced the incidence of significant side-effects. Risk factors for radiation-induced damage include the age at the time of treatment, the total dose delivered and the volume of tissue irradiated. Children undergoing rapid growth (i.e. those <6yrs of age and at puberty) are particularly vulnerable due to the rapid replication of growing tissues (Probert and Parker, 1972). For example, those who have received spinal irradiation often fail to reach their full height due to damage to the growth centres of the vertebral bodies (Shalet et al, 1987) while scoliosis or kyphosis may follow irradiation to one side of the body which results in uneven effects on growing tissues. Thus growth retardation, asymmetrical development and scoliotic deformities are not uncommon. Continued, long term assessment of growth is essential so that rehabilitative actions can be initiated at an early stage should deformity occur.

Osteoradionecrosis, particularly of the mandible, is rarely seen with current therapeutic techniques although the risk is markedly increased in the presence of infection. Assessment and care of this condition are discussed in Chapter 7. Fractures may, occasionally, occur in bones which have previously been irradiated.

REFERENCES

D'Angio GL, Pearson D, 1975, Radiation Therapy. In: Bloom HGJ (Editor), Cancer in Children, Springer-Verlag, Berlin.

Hilderley LJ, 1992. Radiotherapy. In: Groenwald SL, Frogge MH, Goodman M, Yarbro CH, (Editors), Treatment Modalities. Part III from Cancer Nursing Principles and Practice (Second edition), Jones and Bartlett Publishers, Boston.

Holmes S, Dickerson JWT, 1988, Malignant disease: nutritional implications of disease and treatment, Cancer and Metastasis Reviews **6**, 357-381

Jervis HR, Donati M, Stromberg LR, Sprinz H, 1977, Histochemical investigation of the mucosa of the exteriorised small intestine of the rat exposed to x-irradiation, Strahlentherapie, **138**, 326-329.

Mennie AT, Dalley VM, Dinneen L, Collier NOV, 1975, Treatment of Radiation-induced gastrointestinal distress with acetylsalicylic acid, Lancet, ii, 942.

Moore IM, Ruccione K, 1992, Late effects of cancer treatment, In: Groenwald SL, Frogge MH, Goodman M, Yarbro CH (Editors), Manifestations of Cancer and Cancer Treatment Part V from Cancer Nursing: Principles and Practice (Second edition), Jones and Bartlett Publishers, Boston.

Nazarko L, 1995, The therapeutic uses of cranberry juice, Nursing Standard, **9**(34), 33-35.

Probert JC, Parker BR, 1975, The effects of radiation therapy on bone growth, Radiobiology, **114**, 155-162

Ruccione K, Weinberg K, 1989, Late effects in multiple body systems, Seminars in Oncology Nursing, **5**, 6-8.

Shalet SM, Gibson B, Swindell R et al, 1987, Effect of spinal irradiation on growth, Archives of Diseases of Childhood, 62, 461-464.

Sobota AE, 1984, Inhibition of bacterial adherence by cranberry juice: potential use for the treatment of urinary tract infections, Journal of Urology, **131**, 1013-1016.

Zafriri D, 1989, Inhibitory activity of cranberry juice on adherence type 1 and type P fimbriated *Escheria coli* to eucaryotic cells, Antimicrobial Agents and Chemotherapy, **33**(1), 92-98.

CHAPTER 10   EFFECTS ON SEXUAL FUNCTION

Cancer affects all aspects of life and most of those diagnosed with the disease will have concerns about its possible sexual effects as well as those of its treatment (Glasgow et al, 1987; Smith 1989). This is particularly important when it is recognised that cancer is often a chronic disease.

The quality of life of sufferers is of paramount importance thus sexual function, as an important component of the quality of life, takes on increasing relevance. This is true whether or not the individual is undergoing radiotherapy. Yet health care providers often overlook this aspect of care. This may arise for a number of reasons including lack of knowledge or awareness of the impact of the disease and its treatment on sexual function and a general discomfort about discussing such issues with patients.

Clearly the significance of sexual issues varies considerably so that each patient *must* be treated as an individual with his own unique set of fears, worries and needs. Each must be individually assessed and care prescribed on an individual basis.

SEXUAL FUNCTION

The World Health Organisation (1975) describes sexual health as 'the integration of somatic, emotional, intellectual and social aspects of sexual being in ways that are positively enriching and that enhance personality communication and love' thus demonstrating that it incorporates not only the sexual act but also the ability to maintain interpersonal relationships and communicate in a meaningful fashion with significant others.

Psychosocial factors

Optimal sexual function is also dependent on a variety of psycho-social factors (Table 10.1). For example, an adolescent may face a variety of issues in this area including learning to give or receive love, developing relationships with the opposite sex and choosing marital or sexual partner(s) (Woods, 1990). Most adults will focus on sexual activity and gratification within a stable relationship. Sexual activity and interest persist into later life and older adults are no less vulnerable to changes in their sexual functioning (Woods, 1990).

Table 10.1   Psychosocial factors which may affect sexual function

---

Age
Alteration in body image
Reduced self-esteem
Patient's attitudes, beliefs and misconceptions
Anxiety and depression
Role changes
Emotional separation
Physical separation
Availability of a partner
Hospitalisation

Body image and self-esteem are important contributors to the way individuals perceive their sexuality. Developing cancer may produce significant changes in self-esteem, some of which are transient and others permanent. There is little doubt that cancer can exert negative effects on self-esteem whether or not changes in body image are apparent (Folz, 1987). If the patient must also adjust to changes in his physical appearance, his sexual function may be further compromised; this may exacerbate pre-existing anxiety and depression.

Anxiety and depression are commonly observed in cancer patients (e.g. Andersen, 1985) and are also associated with radiotherapy (e.g. Peck and Boland 1977). Clinical depression may be found in between 17 and 25% of all patients hospitalised for the treatment of cancer (Petty and Noyes, 1981). Both anxiety and depression may have significant effects on sexual function.

Similarly, the changing roles within the family may threaten an individual's self-esteem (Johnson, 1986) and, in turn, lead to sexual dysfunction. This should be considered when planning care for affected patients. Thus it is not surprising that many patients feel that they have lost control of their lives. It is not surprising if these effects monopolise the patient's thinking and obliterate his/her desire for a sexual relationship.

The direct effects of cancer on sexual function are dependent on the nature of the disease and the area of the body involved. For example, disease invading the vulva, vagina, cervix, or breast may affect a woman's sexual function and involvement of the testes, urinary tract or penis that of the male. Tactile responsiveness may be affected by neurological involvement and vascular changes may cause physiological dysfunction. Hormonal effects may disturb sexual function through hormonal imbalance.

The clinical manifestations of the disease, such as malaise, fatigue, and physical weakness, may cause a gradual reduction in libido and treatment of the disease may necessitate hospitalisation and physical separation of the patient and his or her partner. Emotional separation can also result from the difficulties associated with both accepting and living with the diagnosis. These effects may combine to make it difficult to establish or maintain an intimate relationship and the stress engendered may cause a fragile relationship to deteriorate.

The partner is also vulnerable to psychological effects that may impact on normal sexual expression. The patient's family have to adjust to many changes and depression and anticipatory grieving lead to an almost constant emotional stress. Anxiety and depression may affect their sexual function and interest. In addition, the physical condition of the patient may cause fears that he is too sick for sexual activity or that he will, in some way, be hurt should sexual activity be attempted. The partner may feel guilty about making sexual overtures to someone who is experiencing the trauma of cancer or its treatment or be concerned that they may catch the disease. For some, the fear that the patient is, somehow, radioactive during their therapy will cause additional anxiety further inhibiting the willingness to engage in sexual activity. Furthermore, a partner may find it difficult to 'switch' roles between that of care-giver and that of sexual partner (Lamb, 1991).

For all these reasons, sexual expression may decrease and may reinforce the patient's belief that he is 'dirty' or 'unclean'. The side-effects of radiotherapy may further decrease the patient's self-esteem through alterations in his body image thus exacerbating sexual difficulties. Fatigue, weakness, nausea and vomiting may also make sexual relationships difficult.

SEXUAL DYSFUNCTION

The sexual response (Table 10.2) in both males and females is initiated by a combination of tactile visual and psychological factors. Psychologically this compromises two main changes - an increase in venous blood flow (vasocongestion) and an increased muscle tension

(myotonia) (Woods, 1990) which are dependent on intact neurological function and an appropriate hormonal environment. According
to Woods (1990), sexual dysfunction may affect the areas of
excitement (desire or interest), arousal (readiness) and orgasm
(release) and may arise, as has been shown, from a variety of external
or internal factors.

Table 10.2   **Cycle of sexual response**

Phase	Female	Male
Excitement (desire or interest) (parasympathetic response)	Lubrication of vagina. Size of clitoris and labia minora increased. Increased sensation felt in clitoris and labia minora. Neuro-muscular tension, breasts enlarge, erection of nipples. Upward movement of uterus.	Erection of penis; testicles drawn up towards body. Erection of nipples. Increase in cardiac and respiratory rate.
Plateau (readiness) (parasympathetic response)	Vagina expands and contractions begin. Clitoris retracts. Uterus draws up further,	Circumference of penis increases. Testes enlarge; lubricating fluid released from Cowper's gland.
Orgasm (sympathetic response)	Uterus contracts, deeper portion of vagina becomes distended. Pelvic thrusts with associated general muscular contractions.	Ejaculation; pelvic thrusts associated with generalised muscular contraction.
Resolution (satisfaction) (parasympathetic response)	Congestion of organs subsides. Uterus and vagina gradually return to pre-excitement state. General release of tension.	Congestion of organs subsides. Loss of erection and return to pre-excitement state. General release of tension.

Note: All of these reactions depend on libido. Progression between stages may
be disrupted by fear, anxiety, anger and lack of privacy. To progress between
stages hope, safety, contentment and privacy are necessary.

DIRECT EFFECTS OF RADIATION

Radiotherapy can cause sexual dysfunction in both female and male
patients. It may cause sterility, impotence, dyspareunia or changes in
body image; its effects on foetal development can be disastrous.

Effects on sexual function

The female

Radiation-induced effects may affect sexuality when either the ovaries or the vagina are included in the treatment field causing a wide range of difficulties.

For example, irradiation of the ovaries may cause temporary or permanent cessation of ovulation resulting in sterility. The long-term effects depend on the dose:time relationship, the woman's age, and the volume of tissue irradiated. Age affects the outcome since the greatest effect of radiation to the ovaries is on the intermediate follicles; when these are significantly damaged permanent sterility may result (Hilderley, 1992). In younger women, the number of oocytes is greater so that the total dose required to produce permanent sterility is higher than is required in the older woman (Yasko, 1983). Because women have fewer oocytes as they approach the menopause, radiation-induced damage is more likely to be permanent (Krebs, 1992). This can be avoided, at least to some extent, by carrying out an oophoropexy (which tucks the ovaries out of the treatment field) which may preserve fertility, even when relatively high doses of radiation have been delivered (Horning et al, 1981)

Whether temporary or permanent sterility is anticipated the menstrual cycle will be disrupted and ovulation is unlikely to occur. Even when this is temporary the normal cycle may not resume for 6-12 months after the completion of treatment. Should subsequent pregnancy be desired it should be remembered that all the ova present in the ovaries were exposed to irradiation so that genetic effects may affect the unborn child (see p146); genetic counselling is essential for such patients, and their partners, although it must also be recognised that many women who have undergone such treatment have successfully given birth to normal infants.

Permanent sterility may result in acute manifestations of the menopause so that the patient may need considerable psychological support and reassurance that sterility affects neither femininity nor sexual drive/desire. Where hormonal replacement therapy is not contraindicated this can be a useful adjunct to treatment.

Other changes may also occur as a result of treatment including a loss of libido, a decrease in vaginal muscle tone and lubrication or vaginal mucositis. Pelvic irradiation may also cause vaginal thinning, dryness and stenosis (Andersen, 1985) leading to dyspareunia. Such problems are likely to persist unless action is taken to prevent or minimise their impact. However, most women experiencing such difficulties are able to overcome them with the use of a vaginal hormone cream (unless this is contraindicated), vaginal dilation and pelvic floor exercises (Shrover et al, 1984).

These effects, when combined with the loss of body hair and the diagnosis of cancer *per se*, may significantly affect the patient's self-image and self-esteem and result in feelings of unattractiveness and undesirability. Encouraging open discussion of the patient's feelings and anxieties is an important intervention. Open communication with her partner is also essential if the patient is to be helped to come to terms with these effects. This is a sensitive area and one in which nurses, in particular, have been shown to be reluctant to initiate discussion (Faulkner and Maguire, 1984). Since this is an area where patients are also loathe to ask questions the opportunity for discussion must be presented; it is then up to the patient if she wishes to take up this opportunity.

Some units prefer to advise that intercourse be avoided during treatment since it is felt that this inhibits healing and increases the risk of secondary infection. However, it is important that the patient is aware that sexual intercourse can, if desired, be continued during the treatment period provided that an effective method of birth control is used and provided the vagina is not affected by mucositis or ulceration (refer to Ch 12 for discussion of vaginal treatments). When the vagina is dry a water-based lubricant, such as K-Y Jelly™, will improve lubrication and prevent discomfort or pain. However, a decrease in libido is to be expected during treatment. Birth control, usually reliant on barrier methods of contraception, must be continued for at least 2 years after treatment to enable hormone levels, particularly oestrogen, to return to normal (Table 10.3).

The male

Men with genitourinary cancers often experience sexual difficulties as a result of the disease itself (Shipes and Lehr, 1982) as well as from its treatment. These may include the ability to attain or to maintain an erection or the inability to ejaculate; at times both difficulties will be present. For example, radiation to the prostrate and the surrounding tissues can cause erection difficulties in 37% of patients (Andersen, 1985), probably a result of the damage to the pelvic vasculature and/or the pelvic nerves (Bachers, 1985). This is usually a permanent condition (Shipes and Lehr, 1982).

Table 10.3   Barrier methods of contraception

Condom	Sheath of latex rubber or PVDC designed to cover the erect penis and contain the semen that is ejaculated. It is advisable to use condoms in conjunction with a spermicide (jelly, foam or cream). A female equivalent is available; this slots into the vagina and functions in a similar fashion.	If the patient is female, it may be helpful if a water-based lubricant (such as K-Y jelly™) is used to prevent trauma to the vaginal mucosa. A small number of people are allergic to either the rubber, the lubricant or the spermicide. In this case, a hypoallergenic brand should be used (e.g. Durex Allergy (London Rubber Company)).
Diaphragm	Shallow dome of rubber or plastic with a metal rim also encased in rubber. The rim may be a flat compressible band (flat spring diaphragm) or a wire-spiral, also covered in rubber (coil spring diaphragm). This fits over the cervix acting as a barrier to prevent sperm reaching the uterus. A spermicide (jelly, foam or cream) should also be used.	A very few women may be unable to use a diaphragm (the vagina may be too long or the cervix too short). A few may be allergic to the rubber or the spermicide although this is less of a problem than it is with condoms.
Cervical cap	Made of rubber/plastic and designed to fit snugly over the cervix to prevent sperm entering the cervical canal. Should be used with a spermicide (jelly, foam or cream).	These devices cannot be used by all women. May be worn continuously, except during menstruation; some suggest that, like the diaphragm, the cap be removed about 6 hours after intercourse.
Vault cap	Dome made of rubber or plastic that fits across the top end of the vagina covering the cervix. Held in place by suction, air being expelled when the cap is pushed into place.	Not as easy to use as the diaphragm but may be useful for those women in whom the vaginal muscles are weak or when the cervix is split, torn or very short.

Radiation may also affect male sexuality when the testes are located in the treatment field leading to impotence, sterility and chromosomal damage the degree and extent being dependent on the dose:time relationship and the volume of tissue included in the treatment field as well as on the physiological and psychological state of the patient.

Various approaches to treatment may expose the testes to radiation-induced damage, even when the testes are not included in the primary treatment field, due to the effects of scattered radiation on the developing sperm. Although the cells of Leydig and mature sperm are relatively radioresistant, the effect of radiation is greatest on the spermatogonia and immature sperm are extremely radio-sensitive. The sperm count does not begin to fall for 6-8 weeks although chromosomal damage may occur giving rise to genetic defects in the offspring (see p146). Depending on the total dose of radiation delivered, infertility may be permanent (Gill, 1985). Alternatively, the reduced sperm count may persist for some time after treatment is completed (6 months-1 year) and the patient is advised to ensure that he does not father a child for at least 2 years after radiotherapy. Effective methods of birth control are, therefore, essential (Table 10.3). When infertility is a matter of particular concern the possibility of sperm banking should be discussed. This involves the cryopreservation (freezing) of semen, and subsequent use for artificial insemination, and can help to overcome this problem for some patients. It must, however, be recognised that this method is only of value if the semen is of good quality since the freezing process may decrease sperm mobility. As a result, although it can be a useful procedure, it does not guarantee success. If sperm banking is unsuccessful artificial insemination by donor (AID) is another option that can be considered.

The cells of Leydig are not affected by irradiation (unless very high doses are used) so that testosterone levels will remain within the normal range and secondary sexual characteristics and sexual drive will be largely unaffected. Ejaculation may, however, be reduced (Schrover et al 1986). Although testosterone levels are largely unaffected, this does not prevent impotence which may be a temporary or permanent effect of treatment. For example, most men treated for prostate cancer using teletherapy will develop either temporary or permanent impotence that may begin 2-3 weeks after treatment begins and may persist for some weeks after its cessation. On occasions, recovery is incomplete. Impotence arises for several reasons including the anxiety, worry, concern and depression that may follow the diagnosis of cancer, the fatigue, lethargy and weakness often associated with radiotherapy and the side-effects of treatment, such as diarrhoea and/or nausea and vomiting. In some cases (e.g. treatment of prostatic cancer), this may arise as a result of damage to the pelvic vasculature or the pelvic nerves (e.g. Herr, 1979; Schrover and von Eschenbach, 1984). When high doses of irradiation are used some of the cells of Leydig may be destroyed so that testosterone levels fall and a decrease in libido occurs. The degree of destruction determines whether impotence is temporary or permanent.

The impact of impotence can be dramatic so that the patient may require a considerable degree of psychological support. If this is a matter of concern to the patient considerable reassurance will be required. When impotence is expected to be permanent testosterone implants may be beneficial and the patient should be referred to the appropriate specialist.

The loss of the ability to engage in sexual intercourse need not, however, prevent the patient from participating in other ways of satisfying his sexual needs so that sexual counselling may be beneficial and help the patient, and his partner, to identify alternative behaviours. For example, hugging and kissing can demonstrate continuing affection. Both partners should be included in counselling to encourage communication of their fears, needs and anxieties. Again the patient may be embarrassed or reluctant to discuss his problems so that carers must make it clear that they understand and give the patient the opportunity to talk if this is what he wishes to do.

General care of the patient suffering from sexual dysfunction

If health care workers are to help the patient to deal with sexual problems they must first be comfortable with their own sexuality and attitudes as well as her counselling skills (Webb, 1987). Contact with the self as a sexual being will be evident to others and will convey comfort to them (Fetter, 1987). If this is not the case help should be sought from a trained counsellor.

Staff must be aware of the sexual implications of the treatment the patient is receiving if appropriate supportive care is to be given. Careful assessment of the patient is required. The literature contains many references to the issue of sexual assessment (e.g. Chapman and Sughrue, 1987); many of these are specific to cancer patients. The following data will provide information on which to base such care:

    1. The usual pattern of sexual activity and the changes

enforced by both the disease and the treatment.

2. The desire and opportunity for sexual activity.
3. The partner's desire and patterns of coping with sexual deprivation.

Such an assessment must be carried out in privacy ensuring that adequate time is available for the patient to express their concerns and anxieties and for discussion to take place. Patients are often glad to be given the opportunity to discuss their sexual concerns and to know that help is available. It is important that the counsellor is non-judgmental and he/she must accept and support the patient's feelings and beliefs about his sexual behaviour. Since nurses have the most enduring relationship with the patient, the task of identifying such problems often falls to this professional group.

It is difficult to identify any way in which the physiological and psychological effects of malignant disease and its treatment can be avoided so that the predominant role of the health care professional is in helping the patient to come to terms with them and to develop appropriate coping mechanisms.

Appropriate assessment, when combined with the nurse's knowledge about both the patient and the sexual effects of the particular tumour and its treatment will help her to predict potential problems and direct her counselling appropriately. Since many of the side-effects of the disease, as well as radiotherapy, may also have an impact on sexuality, through their effects on body image and self-esteem (e.g. alopecia, oral mucositis, diarrhoea, nausea and vomiting), this must also be considered when offering advice for the management of such effects. For example, an awareness of the presence of dypsnoea could lead a carer to ask whether this interferes with the patient's sexual activity. This demonstrates both awareness and understanding and legitimises sexuality as an appropriate area for discussion helping both the patient and his/her partner to cope more effectively with the problems they may face. Since the patient's partner knows and understands the patient he or she should always be involved in discussion with both members of the caring team and the patient. This may facilitate development of a supportive and caring relationship. Most patients will adjust to these effects although the time required for such adjustment is highly variable.

In general, health care professionals need not worry about discussing sexual problems with their patients since many are relieved that their anxiety is recognised. A patient will, in any case, indicate quite clearly whether or not they wish to pursue the discussion and patients generally recognise carers as professionals and quickly become quite comfortable in discussing such matters. The older patient may, however, find such open communication more difficult. Caring and sensitive care can, eventually, overcome such difficulties.

Temporary sexual difficulties are often self-limiting and resolve once the patient has had time to adapt to the presence of the disease and its treatment or to the loss of a part of the body (e.g. breast or testicle) or a change in their usual appearance. Engendering a positive and hopeful outlook is a positive role for health care workers who can also emphasise many of the positive aspects of sexuality by complementing the patient on her beautiful hair or encouraging the use of make up or everyday clothes.

These actions may also help to enhance self-perception of body image and encourage the patient to regain their self-esteem. The partner can play a positive reinforcing role although, it must be recognised, they too may have problems in coping with the changes in their loved one.

For those who are able to maintain sexual activity effective birth control is essential so that contraceptive advice may be required.

GENETIC (TERATOGENIC) EFFECTS

Radiation, even at low doses, can have marked and disastrous effects on foetal development particularly when exposure occurs during the early stages of embryonic development (i.e. the first trimester). Both spontaneous abortion and foetal malformations are common (Krebs, 1992) and, even when the child appears normal, it is possible that they will, later, develop malignant disease, particularly leukaemia, perhaps due to genetic mutation in either the sperm or the ovum. However, foetal damage probably does not occur at doses below 10cGy and is only rarely reported at doses <50cGy (Lamb, 1985). Damage is less likely during the second and third trimesters although growth retardation, sterility and cataracts may occur (Earley, 1983).

Clearly, an undesired pregnancy carrying the risk of genetic abnormality is an added stress for the patient undergoing treatment for cancer and, as sterility may only be temporary, the need for effective birth control cannot be stressed highly enough.

REFERENCES

Andersen BL, 1985, Sexual functioning morbidity among cancer survivors, Cancer, **55**, 1835-1842.

Bachers ES, 1985, Sexual dysfunction after treatment for genito-urinary cancer, Seminars in Oncology Nursing, **1**, 18-24.

Chapman J, Sughrue J, 1987, A model for sexual assessment and intervention, Health Care for Women International, **8**, 87-99.

Earley WC, 1983, Risks of radiation exposure. In: Abrams R, Wexler P (Editors), Medical Care of the Pregnant Patient: Concepts and Management, Little, Brown, Boston.

Faulkner A, Maguire P, 1984, Teaching ward nurses to monitor mastectomy patients, Clinical Oncology, **10**, 383-389.

Fetter MP, 1987, Reaching a level of sexual comfort, Health Education, **18**, 6-8.

Folz AT, 1987, The influence of cancer on the self concept and quality of life, Seminars in Oncology Nursing, **3**, 303-312.

Gill GN, 1985, Endocrine. In: West JB (Editor), Best and Taylor's Physiological Basis of Medical Practice (Eleventh edition), Williams and Wilkins, Baltimore.

Glasgow M, Halfin V, Althausen AF, 1987, Sexual response and cancer, Ca: A Cancer Journal for Clinicians, **37**, 322-332.

Greenberg DB, 1985, The measurement of sexual dysfunction in cancer patients, Cancer, **53** (suppl.), 2281-2285.

Herr HW, 1979, Preservation of sexual potency in prostatic cancer patients after iodine implantation, Journal of the American Geriatric Society, **27**, 17-19.

Hilderley LJ, 1992. Radiotherapy. In: Groenwald SL, Frogge MH, Goodman M, Yarbro CH, (Editors), Treatment Modalities. Part III from Cancer Nursing Principles and Practice (Second edition), Jones and Bartlett Publishers, Boston.

Horning SJ, Hoppe RT, Kaplan HS et al 1981, Female reproductive potential after treatment for Hodgkin's disease, New England Journal of Medicine, **304**, 1377-1382.

Johnson J, 1986, Sexual concerns of the cancer patient, Nursing Republic of South Africa Verpleging, **1**(10), 24-25.

Krebs LU, 1992, Sexual and reproductive dysfunction. In: Groenwald SL, Frogge MH, Goodman M, Yarbro CH (Editors), Manifestations of Cancer and Cancer Treatments. Part V from Cancer Nursing, Principles and Practice (Second edition), Jones and Bartlett Publishers, Boston.

Effects on sexual function

Lamb MA, 1985, Sexual dysfunctioning the gynecologic oncology patient, Seminars in Oncology Nursing, **1**, 9-17.

Lamb MA, 1991, Alterations in sexuality and sexual functioning. In: Baird SB, McCorkle R, Grant M (Editors), Cancer Nursing: A Comprehensive Textbook, WB Saunders Co., London.

Peck A, Boland V, 1977, Emotional Reactions to Radiation Treatment, Cancer, **40**, 180-184.

Petty F, Noyes R, 1981, Depression secondary to cancer, Biologic Psychiatry, **16**, 1203-1220.

Schrover LR, von Eschenbach AC, 1984, Sexual and marital counselling with men treated for testicular cancer, Journal of Sexual and Marital Therapy, **10**, 29-40.

Schrover LR, von Eschenbach AC, Smith DB, Gonzales J, 1984, Sexual Rehabilitation of Urological cancer patients: a practical approach, Ca: A Cancer Journal for Clinicians, **34**, 66-73.

Schrover LR, Gonzales J, von Eschenbach AC, 1986, Sexual and marital relationships after radiotherapy for seminoma, Urology, **27**, 117-123.

Shipes E, Lehr S, 1982, Sexuality and the male cancer patient, Cancer Nursing, **5**, 375-381.

Smith DB, 1989, Sexual Rehabilitation of the Cancer Patient, Cancer Nursing, **12**, 10-15.

Webb C, 1987, Sexual Healing, Nursing Times, **83**, 28 - 30.

Woods NF, 1990, Human Sexuality in Health and Illness, (Third edition), CV Mosby, St Louis.

World Health Organisation, 1975, Education and treatment in Human Sexuality. The Training of Health Professionals. Report of a WHO meeting, Technical Report Series No: 572, WHO, Geneva.

Yasko JM, 1983, Sexual and reproductive dysfunction, In: Yasko JM, care of the Client Receiving External Radiation, Reston Publishing Co., Reston, Virginia.

CHAPTER 11   BONE MARROW SUPPRESSION

Normal bone marrow is essential to life since the cells it produces (erythrocytes, platelets and leucocytes) are responsible for the transport of oxygen and carbon dioxide, for haemostasis and for the maintenance of immune status. Destruction of the bone marrow may, therefore, have significant and far-reaching effects including thrombocytopoenia, leucopoenia and anaemia; when the precursor stem cells are affected, these effects may be prolonged or permanent.

The distribution, structure and cellular composition of the bone marrow varies both with age and with anatomical location (Nias, 1990). In the young individual, active marrow is distributed through all bones while, in the adult, this is carried to the flat bones (sternum, ribs, iliac crest), the vertebrae and the epiphyses of the long bones. Thus, when large volumes of the active bone marrow are included in the treatment field, the effects may be significant, especially when this affects the pelvis or the spine in adults. Other areas of concern include the sternum and ribs and the epiphyses of the long bones.

However, bone marrow suppression following radiotherapy is rarely as severe as that accompanying cancer chemotherapy unless more than 25% of the active bone marrow is included in the treatment field (Table 11.1). This is because the effects of radiation are restricted only to a local area so that substantial amounts of the marrow remain unexposed and are able to compensate for radiation-induced damage, unless the marrow has been damaged by prior therapy. In any case, considerable care is taken to ensure that shielding is provided for as much of the active marrow as is possible and compatible with the aims of treatment.

RADIATION-INDUCED DAMAGE TO THE BONE MARROW

The effects of radiation on the bone marrow are not dissimilar to those of cancer chemotherapy although it is much more damaging to cells in the G_0 phase of the cell cycle. However, unlike chemotherapy, it also negatively affects stromal elements resulting in a disruption of the bone marrow architecture, fibrosis and necrosis (Fliedner et al, 1986). It is the combination of these effects which accounts for the potential long-term consequences of radiotherapy. Residual effects include hypoplasia and/or aplasia of some, or all,

147

Table 11.1   **Percentage of bone marrow affected by normal therapeutic techniques**

Area of irradiation	Estimated percentage of bone marrow affected (%)
Chest wall/lymphatics	15-20
Pelvic	15-25
Abdominal	20-25
Pulmonary/mediastinal	20-25
Mantle	20-50
Cranial	25-45
Total nodal	60-70
Craniospinal	60-75
Total body	100

marrow components. As a result of which patients may be intolerant as a result of which patients may be intolerant of further anti-cancer therapy. It has been estimated that regeneration will not occur after doses of between 3000cGy and 5000cGy (Rubin, 1984; Fliedner et al, 1986).

Radiotherapy may affect erythrocytes, leucocytes and platelets; it is also toxic to lymphocytes, particularly T-cells, when significant portions of the lymphatic system are exposed to radiation (e.g. Blomgren et al, 1981; Du Bois and Serrou, 1981).

COMPLICATIONS OF BONE MARROW SUPPRESSION

Since neither the platelets nor the white blood cells are stored by the body in any significant quantity the effects of bone marrow suppression will be seen first on these cells resulting in thrombo-cytopoenia and leucopoenia. These are major causes of both morbidity and mortality in cancer patients.

Thrombocytopoenia

Since platelets have a rapid cell turnover (life span 8-9 days) they are vulnerable to radiation-induced damage and thrombocytopoenia may be the first sign of bone marrow suppression. However, it may also be due to marrow replacement by tumour cells. Thrombocytopoenia is characterised by bleeding in any site. Petechiae and purpuric areas may appear in the skin or mucous membranes and bleeding from the nose, gums, gastrointestinal or genitourinary tract may occur. The risk of spontaneous bleeding is significant once the platelet count falls below 20 x 10^9/litre (normal range 200-300 x 10^9/litre). Spontaneous haemorrhage may, however, occur when the platelet count is higher than this when other factors intervene to compromise platelet function (e.g. pyrexia, infection). Minor bleeding, such as occult blood in the stools, may occur when the platelet count exceeds 50 x 10^9/litre although such bleeding does not, of necessity, signal the onset of an acute haemorrhage. However, the platelet count is not an absolute indicator of the likelihood of bleeding since this may be affected by many factors including the rate of decline in the platelet count, infection and potential sources of bleeding.

Care of the patient with thrombocytopoenia
The specific care required by patients with bleeding tendencies will vary with the individual, the associated symptomatology and the severity of the condition. There are, however, several common problems and general considerations that are applicable to all affected patients.

All patients suffering from thrombocytopoenia must be closely observed for signs of bleeding. The urine and stools should be routinely tested for the presence of blood; any vomit should also be closely observed. Bleeding may affect the gums or nasal mucosa and epistaxis is common. If menstruation has not been suppressed by treatment, prolonged and heavy vaginal bleeding may occur.

Staff must be alert to the possibility of internal bleeding. Signs and symptoms include pallor, weakness, rapid deep respiration (air hunger), a rapid weak pulse, and hypotension. Mental and neuro-logical status should also be closely monitored (Table 7.1) due to the risk of cerebral dysfunction resulting from bleeding into the brain. Changes in vital signs, such as hypotension and tachycardia, may provide the first indications of spontaneous bleeding.

Measures to prevent bleeding. Preventive measures can be taken to reduce the risk of bleeding. The frequency of invasive procedures should be reduced to a minimum. When subcutaneous or intra-muscular injections are essential, a small gauge needle must be used and gentle pressure applied to the site for several minutes after administration until any bleeding has stopped. Constipation, nausea and vomiting may all increase intracranial pressure and may precipitate bleeding in vulnerable patients. Measures to prevent these problems are essential (Haeuber and Spross, 1991).

Trauma to the body tissues must be avoided so that the patient must be handled gently and, if confined to bed, he should be turned every 1-2 hours to reduce pressure to the tissues. He should be instructed about the importance of avoiding bumps, scratches, and cuts; severe injury can result if he falls out of bed. Use of an electric razor will help to maintain the integrity of the skin and a very soft tooth brush should be used for cleaning the teeth to avoid damaging the gums and mucous membranes. Regular mouthwashes and irrigation will help to maintain oral hygiene.

Patients suffering from thrombocytopoenia must be warned against taking any unprescribed medicine, especially aspirin and aspirin-containing products, since aspirin can both impair platelet function and irritate the gastrointestinal mucosa. Aperients and/or stool softeners may be given to maintain bowel function and prevent constipation and undue straining.

Care during a bleeding episode. The patient should remain in bed during a bleeding episode although, since he may not be experiencing any discomfort, he may find it difficult to remain inactive. At the same time, he may be apprehensive and fearful; his feelings must be acknowledged and reassurance given. Emotional and/or psychological support are an essential part of care. This is particularly true during an acute bleeding episode since this can be very frightening. Rapid intervention, such as the application of an ice pack or direct pressure, may also be required. The patient should not be left alone for long periods since the nurse's presence can provide comfort and reassurance.

Staff should listen to the patient and answer any questions he may have. Platelet transfusions are the treatment of choice when the platelet count falls to less than 100×10^9/litre, when the patient is clinically symptomatic or during episodes of active bleeding. Prophylactic transfusion may be considered when the count falls to 20×10^9/litre (National Institutes of Health, 1989). It must, however, be recognised that this is only a palliative measure and the risk of bleeding will continue until the bone marrow has recovered.

Leucopoenia

Since leucocytes play the major role in the host's resistance to infection, leucopoenia (a deficiency of white blood cells (WBC) below the normal lower limit of $5,000 \times 10^9$/litre) significantly increases the risk of infection in affected patients. This will be exacerbated by malnutrition, the effects of age, recent surgery and drugs, such as corticosteroids (Sarna, 1980). Prevention of infection is, therefore, an essential goal of care.

Care of the patient with leucopoenia

The integrity of the skin and mucous membranes provides an important barrier to infection so that invasive procedures should be kept to a minimum. When these are unavoidable, meticulous aseptic care and close observation are essential, particularly when the patient is also suffering from thrombocytopoenia. The bed-ridden patient is particularly vulnerable due to the risk of pressure sores and hypostatic pneumonia so that regular turning and pressure area care are essential.

When the leucopoenia is marked the patient may be cared for in protective isolation (reverse barrier care) and, ideally, this will be carried out in a single room with filtered air to reduce the risk of air-borne infection. Only sterile equipment and linen are used and staff caring for the patient are screened for possible infection. A clean gown and mask are worn at the bed side and hands must be washed thoroughly under running water before attending to the patient. Only immediate family are allowed to visit and they, too, must wear a gown and mask and avoid physical contact with the patient. This may be difficult for the patient to cope with since isolation can result in significant sensory deprivation.

Nurses and other health care workers must, therefore, be aware of the emotional/psychological effects of isolation and provide comprehensive supportive care. Strategies, such as relaxation and distraction, can be employed and interventions designed to give the patient as much control as possible should be considered.

Oral hygiene is particularly important in the care of these patients and the mouth should be rinsed with normal saline or a mild anti-septic mouthwash every 2 hours (see Ch 7). When the patient is unable to maintain his own oral hygiene the nurse must ensure that she takes over this function for him. A copious fluid intake (2-3000ml/day) will be beneficial. Immune status can be enhanced, to some extent, by means of a high protein, high energy diet. Supplementation with vitamin C may be beneficial.

Routine samples should be taken for bacterial culture; these should include specimens of urine, stools and sputum and swabs from the skin, nose and throat. Swabs are also taken from any suspicious sites, such as an intravenous cannula or urinary catheter.

Bone Marrow Suppression

Anaemia

Anaemia is common in cancer patients (Dutcher, 1986). It is usually relatively mild and so does not require treatment. It may, however, be exacerbated by anticancer therapy, most notably chemotherapy. It may also be associated with nutritional deficiencies (e.g. iron, vitamin B_{12} and folic acid (Hillman and Finch, 1985).

Since the life span of red blood cells is considerably longer than that of leukocytes or platelets (120 days) treatment-induced anaemia may not be seen for some time after treatment and can easily be treated with blood transfusions. Health care professionals must, however, be aware of the signs and symptoms of anaemia so that care can be directed towards its treatment. Regardless of the cause of anaemia the patient will manifest signs and symptoms that are attributable to tissue and organ hypoxia since anaemia decreases the capacity of the blood to transport oxygen.

The severity of the symptoms depends on the degree of anaemia present. Initially, the patient experiences general fatigue, lassitude, and weakness, shortness of breath on exertion and anorexia all of which are non-specific and can be difficult to differentiate from the effects of disease or treatment. Complaints of headache, dizziness and 'tingling' of the extremities are common and diarrhoea or constipation may be present. The mucous membranes and skin become pale. Hypoxia will lead to a fall in the basal metabolic rate so that the patient may feel cold. Palpitations may be present as the heart rate increases in an attempt to reverse the oxygen deficiency. All of these symptoms may be exacerbated in the older individual who may have pre-existing age-related conditions. If the condition is severe, circulatory and renal function may develop causing oedema and, on occasions, angina pectoris due to myocardial hypoxia.

Care of the patient with anaemia

In general, the most effective treatment of anaemia is treatment of the underlying disease, When this is induced by radiotherapy the anaemia itself must be treated.

The care required depends on the severity of the anaemia and is directed towards alleviating the patient's discomfort and preventing any complications. Since the anaemic patient will tire easily he should be encouraged to rest at intervals throughout the day. When the anaemia is severe, bed rest will be required until his haemoglobin level approaches normality. Bed rest necessitates attention to pressure area care and prevention of hypostatic pneumonia and deep vein thrombosis.

A light, varied and digestible diet should be given which is high in energy and protein and which will provide the nutrients necessary for erythropoeisis. This may prove difficult to achieve in the anorexic patient (Ch 6) as a result of which frequent small meals and nutrient dense liquids may prove more acceptable.

Since severe anaemia may cause marked dyspnoea the patient may be more comfortable if he is nursed with the head of the bed elevated or in the sitting position well supported with pillows. Dyspnoea, in addition to anaemia *per se*, may result in a sore and uncomfortable mouth so that oral hygiene becomes an essential part of care.

Blood transfusion may be given to correct anaemia. This may involve administration of either whole blood or packed red blood cells that provide the same oxygen-carrying capacity as whole blood but in a reduced volume of fluid thus reducing the risk of circulatory overload. However, due to the storage time and conditions, the platelets and granulocytes are no longer functional (Widmann, 1985; Pisciotto, 1989).

A patient who is fatigued and lethargic due to anaemia may find it difficult to believe that his symptoms are not due to a progression of his disease particularly if this is also accompanied by a range of radiation-induced side-effects. As a result, he may require a considerable degree of support and reassurance. Nurses must listen to the patient's concerns and provide factual information to convince him that, once his anaemia has been corrected, his condition will improve and he will feel a great deal better.

TOTAL BODY IRRADIATION (TBI)

TBI is used in conjunction with chemotherapy to prepare the patient for bone marrow transplantation in the treatment of haematological malignancies. Its aim is to eradicate all tumour cells prior to the transplant by penetrating those areas that are most resistant to anti-neoplastic drug therapy (e.g. the central nervous system, skin and testes) (Thomas and Fefer, 1985). It, therefore, destroys the stem cells of the bone marrow, remaining leukaemic cells and lymphocytes. Lung shielding is sometimes employed in attempts to decrease the incidence of interstitial pneumonitis or fibrosis.

The patient is exposed to a large, single dose of irradiation

Bone Marrow Suppression

(approximately 10-10.5Gy), over a period of 4-5 hours (or more), a dose that would be lethal if it were not followed by bone marrow transplantation in an attempt to both prevent bone marrow toxicity and effect a cure. Alternatively, TBI may be fractionated over several days. The dose required is carefully calculated to identify that which will be effective and the rate is calculated to cause the least damage to the rest of the body. This is usually achieved by giving a test dose of radiation so as to measure and record the dose variation over the patient's body which will enable the total treatment time required to be calculated. At the same time, this provides the opportunity to familiarise the patient with the treatment room and the procedure facing him and to answer any questions he may have.

The treatment process

Since the patient will have a severely compromised immune status protective isolation is essential; this must be maintained throughout treatment. Where possible this is achieved by means of a laminar air flow filter system. Staff must, therefore, follow strict reverse barrier nursing procedures and all equipment taken into the treatment room must be sterile.

During treatment the patient lies on the treatment table in a position that ensures that his whole body is included in the radiation beam. Although his position is altered in line with the treatment plan, movement is discouraged so that the patient must be made as comfortable as possible using pillows and blankets.

The radiation beam is usually directed at the patient laterally and reversed at the mid-point of treatment. Some units may place the patient in the supine position for part of his treatment. The test doses are repeated before treatment is commenced to verify the calculated dose and necessary exposure time; where necessary corrections are made to the treatment plan.

Since the patient wears few, if any, clothes the treatment room is warmed; this may increase his embarrassment and discomfort. At times, he may be covered with a light blanket.

Care of the patient receiving total body irradiation

Although the patient is often severely debilitated, and may be seriously ill, due to both the side-effects of chemotherapy and his disease, the hope of a cure is often a strong motivating factor in those patients opting for this form of treatment. This means that they are often unrealistically optimistic even though they may be anxious and fearful about their forthcoming treatment. However, it must be recognised that patients can usually tolerate this treatment only once although bone marrow transplantation may be attempted without further irradiation. The prime roles of the nurse are preparation of the patient for his treatment and the provision of psychological support and physical care before, during and after TBI.

Prior to treatment the procedure must be carefully explained and the patient must be told what to expect in terms of side-effects (Table 11.2) and feelings that he might experience during TBI. This may help to reduce his fears and anxieties. Previous assessment will enable identification of measures appropriate for the relief of the patient's pain and discomfort which may be helpful during the treatment period.

An intravenous infusion is usually in position and chemotherapy is usually administered immediately before, or during, TBI according to the treatment protocol. The patient is often sedated throughout treatment. Since the patient must lie still for several hours this may help to overcome some of his discomfort.

Treatment can and should be interrupted for repositioning or symptom relief (e.g. nausea). Such interruptions will also help to relieve the feelings of isolation since this can be a very frightening procedure for the patient. He must be assured that he will be watched constantly via a television monitor; communication via an intercom may be very comforting. The patient must be closely observed for signs of discomfort or other untoward effects.

Although the patient may drink and move around during breaks in his treatment, excessive drinking and movement should be discouraged since this will increase nausea and vomiting. Nausea is, in any case, likely after a dose of approximately 3Gy and can be controlled by appropriate antiemetic therapy. Nausea can be exacerbated by pre-treatment chemotherapy.

Once treatment is completed the patient is returned to the ward. At this stage, he is covered with sterile linen or pyjamas and wears a mask until he is back in the protection of a reverse barrier unit. Patients are often physically exhausted and need to rest although their family may visit, within the restrictions of his requirement for isolation, if this is what he would like. It is often comforting to have some contact with family members after a traumatic period of treatment.

Table 11.2   Side-effects of total body irradiation

Intermediate	Nausea and vomiting	Occurs after a dose of approximately 3Gy. Severity dependant on pre-treatment chemotherapy and level of movement.
	Erythema	Develops during treatment resolving after 24-48 hours.
	Parotitis and pancreatitis	Develop and usually resolve within 24-72 hours of treatment.
	Diarrhoea	Begins rapidly after therapy; subsides within a few days.
	Pyrexia	Develops soon after treatment, resolves within 24 hours.
	Mucositis	Appears within a few days taking some weeks to resolve.
Subacute	Alopecia	Occurs within 2 weeks; regrowth in several months.
	Pneumonitis	Occurs within 2 or more weeks; may result in significant fibrosis.
	Somnolence	May persist for 10-14 days.
Late/chronic	Hyperpigmentation, dryness, peeling, wet desquamation of the skin	Occurs 2-3 weeks after treatment persisting for months.
	Cataracts	Appear long after treatment (20% of patients affected 4 years after treatment); irreversible
	Sterility	May occur months after treatment.
	Growth retardation (children)	May occur in months or years following treatment
	Hepatic/renal damage	May occur months/years after treatment; irreversible.

The immediate side-effects of TBI may be severe and distressing so that health care professionals must be aware of their impact and reassure the patient that some will last only a short time. They may, however, be exacerbated by prior or concurrent chemo-therapy and by bone marrow transplantation itself.

Some patients become febrile immediately after TBI; others develop bilateral parotitis (Hutchison and King, 1983). The chills, nausea and vomiting arising during or shortly after TBI usually resolve within 24 hours; diarrhoea, pancreatitis and parotitis generally last only a few days as does erythema resulting from exposure to radiation. This may, however, be followed by desquamation; wet desquamation may occur several weeks after treatment and persist for some time (Ch 6).

Mucositis, particularly if this is aggravated by concurrent infection, may last for some weeks and alopecia, which usually occurs within 2-3 weeks of treatment, may have significant and long-lasting effects since the regrowth of hair may take several months.

Clearly, the pre-treatment chemotherapy and concomitant drug therapy, may exacerbate these effects and have profound psychological effects on the patient. When this is combined with continuing isolation, due to the risk of infection in the now severely immunosuppressed patient, its effects may be severe so that the care of affected patients is a challenging but rewarding task.

The late effects of radiation-induced damage are rarely major concerns at this stage of treatment; they are, simply, risks that are accepted in the attempt to effect a cure in a patient for whom all other methods of treatment have failed. They may, however, gain increasing importance once long-term survival has been assured.

BONE MARROW TRANSPLANTATION (BMT)

TBI is followed by infusion (transplantation) of bone marrow obtained from a carefully selected donor in an attempt to replace the diseased bone marrow and restore bone marrow function. Immunosuppressive drugs are given to prevent rejection. The process itself is relatively and is not dissimilar to a blood transfusion.

After the transplant the patient must be closely observed to evaluate whether the graft has taken. The focus of care is on provision of optimum support which is heavily reliant on nursing expertise. At this time the patient is at risk of potentially fatal complications (Bearman et al, 1988) which are often insidious in onset. Nursing tasks, such as measurement of vital signs, monitoring of fluid intake and output and body weight, are of extreme importance (Ford and Ballard, 1988).

Bone marrow aspiration is performed weekly and, if the graft is successful, blood cells will begin to develop in the 'new' bone marrow. Until the graft has taken the patient is particularly vulnerable to infection, bleeding and the side-effects of both radiotherapy and chemotherapy. At this stage, opportunistic infections are common as commensal organisms, which are part of the body's normal flora, become pathogenic. Examples include those affecting the mouth, throat and oesophagus (e.g. *Candida albicans* (a fungus) and *Herpes simplex* (a virus) which may exacerbate pre-existing mucositis. It is important to remember that many of these effects are interrelated so that one may cause or exacerbate another; treatment may potentiate such interactions (Storb and Thomas, 1985).

The patient is also at risk of graft-versus-host disease (GVHD) which is unique to BMT patients. This occurs when the transplanted marrow tissue rejects that of the host (Press et al, 1986) since the immunologically competent cells of the graft recognise the patient as 'foreign' and its cells, therefore, react against the host. The onset of GVHD often coincides with engraftment.

GVHD appearing within 3 months of BMT is referred to as acute graft-versus-host disease. When it occurs more than 3 months after transplantation it is called chronic graft-versus-host disease (Graze and Gale, 1979). It primarily affects the skin, liver and gastro-intestinal tract. It is manifested by mild to severe skin reactions that produce a punctate, erythematous rash on the palms of the hands and soles of the feet; if untreated, this progresses to a severe erythema, wet desquamation and blistering and carries the risk of secondary infection. Nausea and vomiting, accompanied by green watery diarrhoea and abdominal pain, may be present. The chronic condition may present in a similar fashion but more often presents as a multi-system disease very similar to the collagen-vascular diseases (Shulman et al, 1980; Jaffee, 1983). Both forms of GVHD can lead to areas of hypo- or hyperpigmentation, loss of elasticity, contractures and ulceration; total body sloughing may occur.

Chronic GVHD may also be accompanied by severe diarrhoea and hepatic failure; it can be fatal. Prolonged immunosuppression, which can help to overcome GVHD, can render the patient particularly vulnerable to viral infections (e.g. *Cytomegalus virus*). Cyclosporin, an immunosuppressive agent, is used to prevent and/or control the condition and sulphur drugs, such as Bactrim™ (Bayer) or Septrin™ (Burroughs-Wellcome), are used to prevent *Pneumocystis carinii* pneumonia (McConn, 1987). Methotrexate may be used, in low doses, to slow the growth of the new marrow and to prevent GVHD and can result in rashes, pruritis, urticaria, photosensitivity and other side-effects. Other therapies used in attempts to prevent GVHD include T-cell-specific monoclonal antibodies (Storb et al, 1986).

Care after bone marrow transplantation

Intensive nursing care is needed during the immediate post-transplant period. Nurses have an important role in helping patients to cope with the uncertainty and in fostering hope (Brack et al, 1988).

They must also plan interventions that give the patient as much control as is possible given the nature of his condition (Haberman, 1988). Thus strategies such as visualisation and distraction can be helpful (Haberman, 1988).

This is a stressful and traumatic period for both the patient and his family due to the range of side-effects he may experience, the uncertainties involved in BMT and the need for prolonged isolation and hospitalisation. This poses a considerable strain on the health care team since not only must they care for the patient but they must also support his family, particularly when one of the family has been the bone marrow donor. These factors may lead both patients and their families to experience a myriad of emotions ranging from hope to despair, anger to joy, anxiety and/or depression (Haberman, 1988). Psychosocial assessment and intervention are, therefore, an essential part of care.

Although appropriate interventions include all those applicable to the patient suffering bone marrow suppression other factors must also be taken into account. These include:

- Reverse barrier care is essential to protect the patient
- Monitoring of body temperature every 4 hours will enable rapid treatment to be initiated when infection is present
- Prophylactic mouthwashes, such as normal saline and hydrogen peroxide, should be given to prevent mucositis and reduce the risk of secondary infection
- Care must be taken to maintain the patient's personal hygiene at an optimal level. Daily baths, using an antiseptic, are recommended
- The perianal area is particularly vulnerable to infection, especially when diarrhoea is present. Meticulous perianal care is essential
- When an intravenous infusion is in progress the insertion site should be inspected daily for signs of infection. A bacteriostatic ointment may be prescribed
- If intestinal mucositis and diarrhoea are severe total parenteral nutrition is essential to offset post-treatment malnutrition.

The success or failure of a bone marrow transplant can usually be determined within 10-20 days. If it is successful the blood cells will begin to develop within the patient's bone marrow and, if remission has been achieved, fewer than 5% of the cells present in the marrow will be blast cells. The polymorphonuclear cells will increase more rapidly than the platelets although both will gradually develop and reach normal levels. Red cells develop more slowly so that it may be several weeks before the haematocrit rises.

As the patient recovers, and is discharged from hospital, continuing support and observation will be required. Bone marrow aspiration and haematological studies are carried out regularly both to ensure that progress is maintained and to detect any relapse as early as possible.

Patients must be advised to stay away from crowds and from any individual (even a family member) suffering from any form of infectious disease for 3-6 months after discharge from hospital since their immune function will be compromised for some time following even a successful bone marrow transplant.

Although total body irradiation is now curing patients who were otherwise incurable (McElwain, 1985), provided that the bone marrow is replaced with marrow from a healthy donor (bone marrow transplantation), it is a procedure not without risk. The nurse has a vital role to play in preparing patients beforehand and in helping them to adjust both physically and psychologically to the changes that take place. Although it is a traumatic experience it is one that gives the patient a better chance to live a normal life.

WHOLE BODY IRRADIATION

Whole body or hemi-body irradiation are occasionally employed in treating those with other malignant diseases. For example, TBI may be used to treat chronic lymphocytic leukaemia (Hilderley, 1992) when it is usually used in a fractionated cycle of 5cGy for 10 days (i.e. 50cGy) repeated, at two week intervals, to a total dose of 150cGy.

Hemi-body irradiation may be used to treat the pain and/or pathological fractures associated with bone metastases, especially when these are widespread. Gilbert et al (1977) have shown that radiotherapy can relieve bone pain in the majority (73-96%) of patients (Ch 13).

REFERENCES.

Bearman SI, Appelbaum FR, Buckner CD et al, 1988, Regimen-related toxicity in patients undergoing bone marrow transplant, Journal of Clinical Oncology, **6**, 1562-1568.

Blomgren H, Baal E, Jarstrand C et al, 1981, Effect of external radiation therapy on the peripheral lymphocyte subpopulation, In: DuBois B, Serrou B, Rosenfeld C (Editors), Immunopharmacologic Effects of Radiation Therapy, Raven Press, New York.

Brack G, LaClave L, Blix S, 1988, The psychological aspects of bone marrow transplants: a staff perspective, Cancer Nursing, **11**, 221-229.

DuBois B, Serrou B, 1981, Effects of ionising radiation on cell-mediated immunity in cancer patients, In: DuBois B, Serrou B, Rosenfeld C (Editors), Immunopharmacologic Effects of Radiation Therapy, Raven Press, New York.

Dutcher JP, 1986, Platelet and granulocyte transfusions in cancer patients. In: Ray PK (Editor), Advances in Immunity and Cancer Therapy, Springer-Verlag, New York.

Fliedner TM, Northdruft W, Clavo W, 1986, The development of radiation late effects to the bone marrow after simple and chronic exposure, International Journal of Radiation Biology, **49**, 35-46.

Ford RC, Ballard B, 1988, Acute complications after bone marrow transplantation, Seminars in Oncology Nursing, **4**, 15-24.

Gilbert HA, Kagan AR, Nussbaum H et al 1977, Evaluation of radiation therapy for bone metastases: pain relief and quality of life, American Journal of Roentgenology, **129**, 1095-1097.

Graze PR, Gale RP, 1979, Chronic graft-versus-host disease: a syndrome of disordered immunity, American Journal of Medicine, **60**, 611- 620.

Haberman MR, 1988, Psychosocial aspects of bone marrow transplantation, Seminars in Oncology Nursing, **4**, 55-59.

Haeuber D, Spross JA, 1991, Alterations in protective mechanisms: haematopoeisis and bone marrow depression, In: Baird SB, McCorkle R, Grant M (Editors), Cancer Nursing. A Comprehensive Textbook, WB Saunders Co., London.

Hilderley LJ, 1992. Radiotherapy. In: Groenwald SL, Frogge MH, Goodman M, Yarbro CH, (Editors), Treatment Modalities. Part III from Cancer Nursing: Principles and Practice (Second edition), Jones and Bartlett Publishers, Boston.

Hillman RS, Finch CA, 1985, Red Cell Manual (Fifth edition), FA Davis Co., Philadelphia.

Hutchinson MM, King AH, 1983, A nursing perspective on bone marrow transplantation, Nursing Clinics of North America, **18**, 511-522.

Jaffee BD, 1983, Chronic graft versus host disease as a model for scleroderma, Cellular Immunology, **77**, 11-20.

McConn R, 1987, Skin changes following bone marrow transplantation, Cancer Nursing, **10**, 82- 84.

McElwain TJ, 1985, The Treatment of Cancer. In: Davis AJS, Rudland PS (Editors), Medical Perspectives in Cancer Research, Ellis Horwood Ltd., Chichester.

National Institutes of Health, 1989, Transfusion alert. Indications for use of Red Blood Cells, Platelets and Fresh Frozen Plasma, Publication No: 89-2974a, Washington DC.

Nias AHW, 1990, An Introduction to Radiobiology, John Wiley and Sons, Chichester.

Pisciotto PT (Editor), 1989, Blood Transfusion Therapy. A physician's Handbook, American Association of Blood Banks, Arlington, Virginia.

Press OW, Schaller RT, Thomas ED, 1986, Bone marrow transplant complications. In: Toledo-Pereya LH (Editor), Complications of Organ Transplantation, Marcel Dekker, New York.

Rubin P, 1984, Late effects of chemotherapy and radiation therapy: a new hypothesis, International Journal of Radiation Oncology, Biology and Physics, **10**, 5-34.

Sarna G, 1980, Oncologic emergencies and urgencies: recognition and treatment. In: Sarna G (Editor), Practical Oncology, Houghton-Mifflin, Boston.

Shulman HM, Sullivan KM, Weiden PL, 1980, Chronic graft versus host syndrome in man. A long term clinicopathologic study of 20 Seattle patients, American Journal of Medicine, **69**, 204-217.

Storb R, Thomas ED, 1985, Graft-versus-host disease in dog and man. The Seattle experience. In: Moller G (Editor), Immunological Reviews No 88, Munksgaard, Copenhagen.

Storb R, Deeg HJ, Farewell V et al, 1986, Marrow transplantation for aplastic anaemia: Methotrexate alone compared to a combination of methotrexate and cyclosporin for prevention of acute graft-vs-host disease, Blood, **68**, 119-125.

Thomas ED, Fefer A, 1985, Bone marrow transplantation. In: DeVita VT, Hellman S, Rosenberg SA (Editors), Cancer: Principles and Practice of Oncology (Second edition), JB Lippincott, Philadelphia.

Widmann FK (Editor), 1985, Technical Manual, American Association of Blood Banks, Arlington, Virginia.

CHAPTER 12   BRACHYTHERAPY

The term 'brachytherapy' describes internal radiation therapy in which a radioisotope is used to provide a high dose of radiation to a tumour or the tumour bed and a rapid fall-off in the dose received by adjacent normal tissues (Hilderley and Dow, 1991). It may be the sole method of treatment or be used in combination with teletherapy. It is designed to improve local control of the disease, preserve function and reduce the damage incurred by associated normal tissues. Although it was, initially, developed as a treatment for gynaecological cancers it is now used to treat cancers at a variety of sites (Table 12.1).

Table 12.1   **Some applications of brachytherapy**

Method of application	Disease	Radioisotope
Sealed sources		
Intracavity	Cervical cancer	Radium-226, Caesium-137
		Radium-226, Caesium-137
	Uterine cancer	
Interstitial	Breast cancer	Iridium-192, Yttrium-90
		Iodine-125, Gold-198,
	Prostatic cancer	Radium-226, Iridium-192,
	Head and neck tumours	Caesium-137
Surface/mould therapy	Basal cell tumours	Radon-222
Unsealed sources		
Oral	Thyroid cancer	Iodine-131
Intravenous	Polycythaemia rubra vera	Phosphorus-32
	Bone pain (skeletal metastasis)	Strontium-90
Intrapleural instillation	Malignant effusion	Gold-198
Intraperitoneal instillation	Ovarian cancer, ascites	Phosphorus-32

Substances with a short half life (hours or days) are used as permanent implants; those with a longer half life (weeks/years) must be removed once the specified dose has been delivered.

Brachytherapy may involve:

1. Contact therapy used, for example, in treatment of the skin.
2. Intracavity treatment when the radioactive source is placed in a body cavity. This is used primarily in the treatment of gynaecological tumours (e.g. cancer of the cervix or uterus).

3. Interstitial therapy which entails implantation of radioactive materials into the tissues (e.g. buccal cavity or breast).

4. Systemic treatment when radioisotopes are administered orally or intravenously (e.g. ^{131}I used to treat thyrotoxicosis or ^{32}P to treat polycythaemia rubra vera).

RADIOBIOLOGY AND BRACHYTHERAPY

The principles of radiobiology were described in Chapter 3. However, when radiation is delivered continuously - as in brachytherapy - the effects on body cells may differ. The radiobiological principles of repair, repopulation, redistribution and re-oxygenation have different implications when this method of treatment is employed.

Repair: Since brachytherapy involves a continuous dose of radiation, sublethal damage is likely to accumulate while repair is inhibited.

Redistribution/repopulation: Redistribution of cells occurs after delivery of each fraction of external radiation (see p29). However, cells are often blocked in the G_2 phase of the cell cycle; continuous radiation will block a greater percentage of cells in G_2. Although cell proliferation may continue, new cells will in turn, be blocked and so vulnerable to radiation-induced damage. In other words, continuous low-dose radiation redistributes a significant proportion of the cell population into G_2 increasing its radiosensitivity and augmenting the radiation effect.

Re-oxygenation: Continuous low-dose radiation reduces the need for oxygen within a tumour during therapy (Hall, 1978; Glicksman, 1987). The effect of brachytherapy may, therefore, be more damaging to hypoxic cells than external beam therapy.

DOSE RATES

Brachytherapy is, typically, delivered at low-dose rates (LDR) (Table 12.2) when patients may be cared for on the wards as long as lead shielding is available and working practices are well controlled (see below). At higher dose rates (HDR), patients must be cared for in a shielded (protected) environment, usually a single lead-lined room. Most LDR therapy involves treatment over several days given in one, or possibly two, fractions (Aird and Williams, 1993). Although HDR therapy requires shorter treatment periods, several fractions may be given.

Table 12.2   Conventional doses for brachytherapy
(Aird and Williams, 1993)

Intracavity therapy	13-17Gy per day (50-70cGyh⁻¹)
Interstitial therapy	7-20Gy per day (30-90cGyh⁻¹)

Intracavity therapy $\quad$ 13-17Gy per day (50-70cGyh^{-1})

Interstitial therapy $\quad$ 7-20Gy per day (30-90cGyh^{-1})

SEALED AND UNSEALED SOURCES

Sources used in brachytherapy may, as shown in Chapter 4, be sealed or unsealed. A sealed source is one in which a solid radioisotope is held within an inert container which provides minimum attenuation of the irradiation. The radioactive material is encapsulated so that it cannot be 'lost' or damaged by any foreseeable degree of chemical or physical stress (Aird and Williams, 1993).

Unsealed sources are contained within a solution or a colloidal suspension; they are, therefore, in liquid form. This method of treatment is also known as systemic radionuclide therapy (Flower and Chittenden, 1993).

RADIATION SAFETY

As shown in Chapter 2, the Ionising Radiations Regulations (1985) state that the maximum permissible dose of radiation for whole body occupational exposure is 50mSv per calendar year (see Table 2.3). In establishing such regulations, factors such as age, occupational and non-occupational exposure and exposure of critical organs are taken into account. This is supplemented by the requirement that exposure is kept as low as reasonably achievable (the ALARA principle). This means that all unnecessary exposure should be avoided thus providing an overwhelming argument in favour of using afterloading techniques (Ch 4). However, as has been shown, such techniques require complex and sophisticated equipment that may not be available in all units. Despite its undoubted value, afterloading is not essential and well controlled working practices, combined with the use of appropriate shielding, can maintain the exposure of all staff involved below the acceptable occupational dose limits (Easson and Pointon, 1985).

The principles of time, distance and shielding (Ch 2) provide the best guidelines for the safety of staff and serve as the basis for safe and efficient patient care. There is no reason why a patient undergoing brachytherapy should not receive adequate care although efforts must be made to protect other patients and staff by alerting them to the risks associated with radiation exposure. It is important to remind staff that the longer the time of exposure the greater is the likelihood of absorption of radiation.

Unnecessary or excessive exposure must be avoided so that 'rotation' of nursing staff is advisable. The importance of minimising exposure must be stressed since radiation cannot be seen or felt and there is no physical discomfort to 'remind' staff of the need to do so. Since radiation can damage a developing foetus (teratogenic effects) (Ch 10) pregnant staff and/or visitors should not attend to the patient whilst the radioactive source is in place. These concerns may cause significant anxiety in staff involved and they may themselves need reassurance and emotional support. They may be fearful of the effect that radiation may have on them. Such fears predominantly arise from misunderstandings and misconceptions of radiation and inadequate knowledge of radiobiology. Appropriate support and education is essential in helping them to overcome their fears as these may be transmitted to the patient and decrease the quality of care.

Restricting the time spent with the patient need not, however, mean 'running away' after giving rapid and ineffective care. What it does mean is that each procedure must be carefully planned and well-organised so that all necessary equipment is prepared and assembled away from the bed side or behind shielding. This not only reduces staff exposure but also lessens the appearance of undue haste thereby reducing the patient's feeling of ostracism. His sense of well-being can also be enhanced not only by ensuring that all his needs are met but also that he is able to reach all the items he is likely to require. A call bell must be available.

Shielding: The type of shielding employed depends on the type of radiation involved and its power of penetration (Ch 3). The maximum thickness that particulate radiation can penetrate (the range) varies (Ch 2). For example, the penetration of α particles is very poor and a few sheets of paper are sufficient to stop them. Thus α particles are not an external hazard. Similarly, the range of β particles is limited and they cannot penetrate the outer layers of the skin. Gamma rays, however, have much greater powers of penetration and a proportion can pass through almost any shield although the percentage of radiation that can penetrate decreases as the thickness of the shielding increases. Thus, it should be noted that lead aprons are not good protection against γ rays since the lead is not thick enough to prevent their penetration (Burns, 1982) and the weight of the apron may mean that it takes longer to complete the task. It also gives the 'illusion' of safety and, therefore, encourages carelessness.

Distance: Safety can be improved if it is remembered that radiation intensity decreases by the square of the distance between the source and the nurse so that a nurse standing 2 metres from the radioactive source receives only and at 4 metres only of the exposure she would receive when standing just 1 metre away. (Figure 12.1).

Figure 12.1   **The inverse square law**

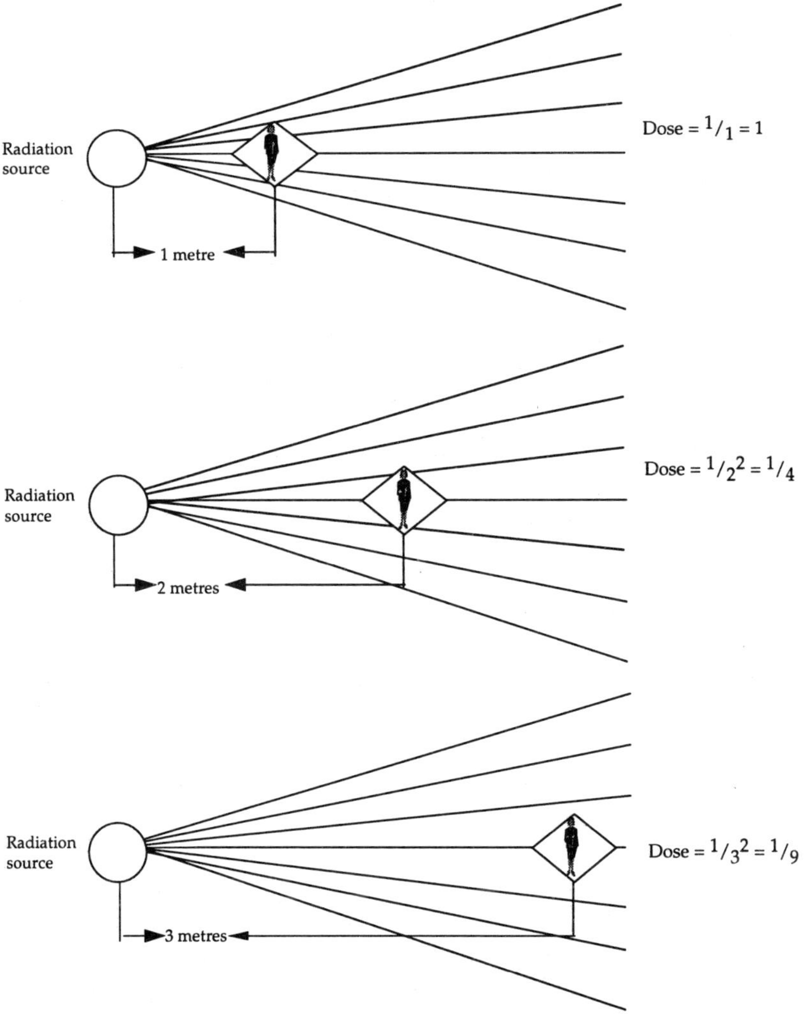

Radiation source

1 metre

Dose = $^1/_1 = 1$

Radiation source

2 metres

Dose = $^1/_2{}^2 = ^1/_4$

Radiation source

3 metres

Dose = $^1/_3{}^2 = ^1/_9$

Control of the working environment
Where afterloading techniques are not employed the exposure of both staff and visitors must be limited as far as possible (ALARA). A typical time limitation on nursing procedures, in close proximity (i.e. at a distance of about 0.5 metres) to a patient receiving brachytherapy for cancer of the cervix, should be in the region of 10 minutes per 9 hour working day (Aird and Williams, 1993). It must be remembered that radiation exposure is cumulative and that it is the total exposure over time that is important.

The number and position of all radioactive sources must be ascertained; regular checks should be made to ensure that they are still in position. A shielded container should be placed near the patient's bed so that, if a source is accidentally displaced, it can be transferred to the container, using long-handled forceps. The time when this occurred should be noted and the Radiation Officer must be called. The intended time of removal of the sources must be noted and a check made to ensure that the exact number of sources has been removed. The patient must be checked with a portable radiation detector to ensure that no sources have been left *in situ*. If a source is missing the actions outlined below should be followed.

All dressings and excreta should be monitored prior to disposal to ensure that they do not contain radioactive sources (using a Geiger-Muller counter) and all rubbish bins, etc. coming from a ward in which brachytherapy is employed, should be tested for radioactivity.

Loss or damage to a sealed source
Clear instructions should exist for dealing with situations in which a radioactive source is lost or mislaid. If a source is lost, no items must be removed from the vicinity of the patient and the Radiation Officer must be called without delay. A thorough search must be instigated using an appropriate radiation detector. When a source is spilled the guidelines presented on in Chaper 2 (p23) should be followed.

IMPLICATIONS FOR PATIENTS
Management of patients undergoing brachytherapy is, inevitably, concerned with ensuring maximum safety of the patient, the health care team and all others coming into contact with the patient (e.g. domestic staff, relatives and friends) while, at the same time, providing optimal care, comfort and reassurance for the patient (see Table 12.3). The patient's fears and anxieties about becoming 'radioactive' should

Table 12.3 Recommendations for the safe use of ionising radiations (sealed sources)

---

1. A monitoring device must be worn at all times when on duty.

2. The patient's bed must be clearly marked with a notice bearing the standard symbols for as long as the source is *in situ.*

3. The time taken for nursing procedures must be reduced to a minimum so that unnecessary time is not spent in close proximity to the patient. Routine procedures should be postponed until the source is removed.

4. Ideally the patient will be nursed in a single room. When cared for on a ward, their bed should be at least 2.5m from adjacent beds and appropriate shielding must be available.

5. Lead shielding must be available for protection of staff.

6. All linen, dressings and other waste products must be monitored before disposal, using a Geiger counter. This ensures that no radio-active sources are accidentally disposed of. Monitoring should be carried out away from the bed side to eliminate background radioactivity. Nurses must be sure that they are familiar with the appearance of the sources in use.

7. When a source is dislodged both the clinician and physicist must be informed. No attempt should be made to replace the source; it should, instead, be placed in a lead container using long handled forceps.

8. Visitors are allowed only the restricted exposure displayed on the warning notice; children and pregnant women must not be allowed to visit.

---

be confronted and can often be overcome by appropriate patient education and counselling prior to the start of the treatment. The patient must be warned that he will be cared for in isolation for as long as the source is in place. The nurse will work quickly and remain with the patient for only long enough to carry out essential activities although she will always be available when required. The patient must, therefore, be encouraged to do as much as possible for himself.

Patients bearing radioactive sources should not leave the treatment room or ward without the prior approval of the radiation physicist. In summary, those with temporary implants cannot leave the hospital until the source has been removed. For those with permanent implants the rules applied apply equally to those receiving treatment with unsealed sources and are dependant in the method of transport. Other factors that determine whether a patient can be discharged include: the radionuclide involved, the residual radioactivity in the patient and his home circumstances. For example, a patient treated with a β emitter (such as ^{192}Ir) will present no external radiation hazard while a patient bearing a source which emits gamma rays (e.g. ^{42}P) will present a much greater hazard and must remain in hospital until the residual radioactivity has fallen to an appropriate level.

TREATMENT WITH SEALED SOURCES

Each solid radioisotope has unique physical features on which its clinical usefulness depends. In addition, the use of particular sources often depends on the preferences of the physicians concerned. The following discussion outlines just some of the potential uses of particular radioisotopes.

Intracavity implants involve insertion of a radioactive source into a body cavity; one of two techniques may be employed. Firstly, both the applicators and the source may be inserted under general anaesthesia. Alternatively, an afterloading technique may be used in which the applicators are inserted in the operating theatre but the source is not implanted until the patient has returned to the 'safety' of the ward (see Ch 4). In both cases, the site of the applicator(s) is checked by X-ray.

Caesium-137 implants are used in the treatment of cervical, uterine and vaginal tumours as described in Ch 4. They emit both β particles and γ rays. Patients are admitted 12-48 hours before treatment and a full medical and nursing history is taken; the procedure is explained to the patient. A consent form must be signed before treatment commences.

In addition to the usual pre-operative preparation, concern must be directed towards the emotional well-being of the patient who may require considerable psychological support particularly with regard to perceived body image, sexuality and possible sterility (particularly in the pre-menopausal woman) all of which may lead to depression and anxiety. Sensitive nursing can help to overcome such effects by helping the patient to explore their feelings and express their fears. Reassurance that sexual activity may be resumed 3-6 weeks after treatment, advice on the use of vaginal dilators and lubricants to prevent atrophy of the vagina, and painful, dry intercourse, may also be helpful.

Specific bowel preparation and a low residue diet for several days pre-operatively will ensure that the colon is empty before treatment commences. This will both aid patient comfort and prevent bowel movements during therapy when care is directed towards preventing displacement of the source(s). A urinary catheter is usually inserted in theatre to prevent movement on to, and off, bedpans during the treatment period. A high fluid intake should be encouraged to promote drainage.

Insertion of the applicators is carried out under general anaesthetic with the patient in the lithotomy position. The vulva, perineum and vagina are cleaned and dilators are passed to ensure no pyometra is present. The sterile applicators and sources are then inserted and the attached strings (needed to facilitate removal) are brought to the surface. A pack is inserted both to keep the sources in position and to reduce the rectal dose. A Geiger counter probe is inserted into the rectum to check the dose; if this is too high the vagina is re-packed or the source changed. The strings may be strapped to the leg or tucked into the vagina; a T bandage or sanitary pad is applied. On return to the ward the patient must remain on bed rest with only 2 pillows throughout treatment; this is essential to avoid displacement of the sources. Sedation and/or analgesia may be needed to maintain comfort.

Observations are made of the patient's temperature and perineal pads at least 4 hourly to monitor for the occurrence of infection and to assess the amount of bleeding or drainage; when this is heavy or unusual the physician must be notified promptly. Possible complications are shown in Table 12.4.

The sources and applicators are carefully removed after the prescribed dose has been administered; the urinary catheter is also removed at this time. Sedation and/or analgesia may be prescribed prior to removal and should be given one hour beforehand. Alternatively, Entonox (50% oxygen, 50% nitrous oxide) is an effective relaxant.

Two nurses should check the time, number and type of applicators before removal is undertaken. The patient should then be placed in the dorsal position with the knees apart. The nurse, working behind lead screens, should then check for and, where necessary, remove any sutures before removing the vaginal packing. The strings of each applicator are identified and the last applicator inserted is removed first.   Each source is removed by gentle traction and placed immediately in a pre-prepared lead container. On completion, two nurses must check that the correct number and type of applicator have been removed.

Table 12.4   Complications of gynaecological applicator
                          treatment

A. DURING TREATMENT	Action
1. Patient may have a bowel action	Check position of the source.

2. Pyrexia
May be due to:
  a. Physiological breakdown of the
    tumour
  b. Chest or urinary tract infection
  c. Reaction to proflavine packing
  d. Pelvic inflammation
  e. Peritonitis due to perforation of the uterus
    (extremely rare)
	Give aspirin or other anti-pyrexial
	drugs

3. Patient may remove applicator	Inform physician and radiation physicist

B. AFTER TREATMENT		
Early	Diarrhoea (transient)	Bland diet, antidiarrhoeal medication
	Urinary frequency and dysuria	Ensure copious fluid intake
	Haemorrhage	Report to physician
	Deep vein thrombosis	Report to physician
Late	Vaginal adhesions, stenosis	Prophylactic use of vaginal dilators and lubricants
	Pyometra	Antibiotic therapy
	Rectal damage - stricture, stenosis, ulceration and haemorrhage	Symptomatic treatment

The patient may get out of bed once she, the bed linen and other waste have been monitored. Vaginal douches may be prescribed after removal of the implant although some physicians believe that this may increase the risk of ascending infection.

The patient is usually discharged on the day after removal of the implant. Such treatment is usually administered on two or three occasions, 2-3 weeks apart although individual physicians may adopt different approaches. Vaginal dilators and lubricants may be prescribed the use of which will stretch the area and prevent fibrosis of the vaginal canal.

Other sealed sources: Iridium-192 seeds or, more commonly, wires, may be used to treat Stage 1 or Stage 11 breast disease when they are used in conjunction with lumpectomy and axillary node dissection to replace the previously used radical mastectomy. Such implants undergo β decay and are usually inserted twice the first insertion following immediately after initial surgery and second 2-3 weeks later.

This treatment, particularly when followed by teletherapy and/or chemotherapy, ensures a good cosmetic result and is effective in controlling or curing the disease. They are also used to treat tumours of the tongue and as a high dose rate source for a variety of intracavity and interstitial treatments.

Although general radiation safety principles must be upheld, few specific nursing interventions are required. Care is directed towards support, reassurance and education. A clean, dry dressing is applied to the insertion site which is observed for signs of infection; antibiotic creams may be prescribed if the wounds become infected.

Prostatic cancer may be treated by use of ^{125}I seeds which are surgically, and permanently, inserted. Since ^{125}I seeds are of relatively low strength and penetration the radioactivity reaching the skin surface is low so that the radioactivity emitted by the patient is low. As a result, he is usually discharged 5-6 days after surgery after the room, urinary drainage bag and the patient himself have been carefully checked for radioactivity.

No specific pre-operative preparation is required. A urinary catheter is inserted at the time of operation and the patient will remain on bed rest for the first 4-5 postoperative days. Pain may be experienced at the site of the surgical wound particularly when the prostate has been approached through the abdomen. Dysuria is common and may last for up to 6 months following this procedure.

SYSTEMIC RADIATION: UNSEALED SOURCES

Radioactive substances may be administered internally via the intravenous or oral route or instilled directly into a body cavity. The use of unsealed sources is a small but rapidly growing approach to radiation therapy. Their use is always associated with a greater radiation hazard than the use of sealed sources both during administration and during the immediate post-treatment period.

Two groups of radioisotopes may be used: the local non-absorbable substances instilled directly into a body cavity to treat a localised area (e.g. ^{198}Au) and the selective uptake isotopes (e.g. ^{131}I). As with other forms of radiotherapy, the dose of radiation that can be delivered to the tumour, is limited by the maximum dose that can be tolerated by normal tissues.

Using systemic therapy, the dose-limiting organ is often the bone marrow so that, if there is a risk of bone marrow suppression, bone marrow may be harvested before therapy for late regrafting. If the isotope is taken up by the liver, this could result in radiation hepatitis and, since many radioisotopes are excreted in the urine, the bladder is also vulnerable to radiation-induced damage. Patients must be hydrated, using intravenous fluids, to reduce the dose delivered to the bladder mucosa

The hazards associated with both types of radioisotope are similar relating to accidental spillage, and leakage from the injection site. Late hazards, however, vary depending on the isotope used and the route of administration. The isotopes most commonly used for this method of treatment are colloidal gold-198, phosphorus-32 and iodine-131.

Gold-198 and phosphorus-32 may both be used in the treatment of malignant pleural effusions or ascites when they are inserted into the appropriate body cavity. Fluid is first removed from the pleural or peritoneal cavity before the liquid radioisotope is instilled into the cavity. Frequent changes of position should be encouraged to promote an even distribution of the radioactive source.

Both radioisotopes may be given systemically in the treatment of polycythaemia rubra vera. Iodine-131 is primarily used to treat malignant disease of the thyroid gland and is most commonly used as an adjunctive therapy following surgical removal of the tumour. When metastatic disease is present the dose may be repeated every 3-4 months.

When colloidal suspensions are used, as described above, a small amount of leakage from the body cavity is to be expected during treatment; this may concentrate in the lymph nodes (Flower and Chittenden, 1993). This may be beneficial in the treatment of malignant disease; it is less desirable when treating other conditions.

In all cases of treatment with unsealed radioactive sources strict isolation must be maintained for the duration of the half life of the isotope involved. General safety precautions must be taken to protect both the staff and other patients.

When pleural effusions or ascites are being treated specific safety measures relate primarily to careful handling and disposal of dressing materials. Dressing changes are carried out wearing rubber gloves and using long-handled forceps and discarded dressings must be monitored for radioactivity prior to disposal; contaminated dressings must be disposed of by the radiation safety officer. Contamination of dressings can be reduced by minimising/preventing leakage around the instillation site by use of occlusive dressings and, where appropriate, a pressure bandage.

Patients undergoing such treatment are usually very ill requiring nursing care directed towards pain relief, prevention of pressure sores, and general hygiene as well as supportive psychological or emotional care. Regular changes of position will not only relieve pressure and enhance comfort but will also help to ensure complete distribution of the radioactive isotope to all areas of the cavity.

Those undergoing treatment with ^{131}I require similar care. Uptake of the isotope is almost exclusively limited to thyroid tissue: excretion is by means of the urine, sweat and saliva and, when this has been administered orally, vomit. Thus, when a patient is incontinent of urine he should be catheterised before the source is administered. All linen must, therefore, be monitored prior to its removal from the patient's room. Patients are hydrated using intravenous fluids for at least the first 24 hours.

Patients undergoing treatment with ^{131}I are allowed no visitors in the first 24 hours following administration after which visitors are permitted but the length of the visit is restricted to the time indicated on the warning notice. The visitor must be instructed to sit several feet from the patient and to avoid physical contact with either the patient or his bed linen. A chair that has not been used by the patient should be provided.

When treatment with ^{198}Au is undertaken visiting is permitted provided visitors remain in the vicinity of the patient for no longer than the time indicated on the warning notice.

In all cases of systemic therapy, the patient must give his written consent to treatment and must also agree to remain in hospital until it is deemed safe for him to be released; discharge is planned by the Radiation Protection Officer in conjunction with the physician (see earlier discussion). No patient is discharged until the amount of radio-activity in his body has fallen below a clearly defined level. The rate of decline depends not only on the half life of the isotope involved but also on the dose administered and the rate of excretion from the body.

Discharge also depends on the type of transport and the length of the journey to be undertaken. Careful instruction is required regarding use of public transport, avoiding both pregnant women and children and separate sleeping arrangements although these restrictions are required for only a short period until the radioactivity carried by the patient has decayed.

TREATMENT WITH RADIOLABELLED ANTIBODIES

Although treatment with radiolabelled antibodies is not yet consistently successful this is an area of growing interest due to the possibility of developing targeted therapy. It is believed that this may, in time, increase therapeutic efficacy by improving localisation and retention of drugs and/or radioisotopes thus reducing toxicity to normal tissues (Baldwin and Byers, 1987). To date, however, a number of problems exist. For example, it is essential that the antibodies employed show good immunoreactivity with the tumour and as little cross-reactivity with normal tissues as possible (Flower and Chittenden, 1993) (i.e. a monoclonal antibody).

However, studies show that only a proportion of the antibody dose actually localises in the tumour while a significant amount remains in the circulation or the reticulo-endothelial system (Morgan and Foon, 1986). Side-effects are, therefore, common and include fever, chills, flushing, rashes and urticaria, hypotension, and nausea and vomiting (Oldham and Smalley, 1983; Dillman, 1988). Bone marrow suppression may occur and, after repeated treatments, allergic reactions are likely due to the foreign antibody (Flower and Chittenden, 1993). In addition, poor tumour vascularity may mean that the antibody may not reach all of the tumour. Nonetheless, advances in medical knowledge, understanding and technology may yet allow this method of treatment to be further developed.

REFERENCES

Aird EG, Williams JR, 1993, Brachytherapy. In: Williams JR, Thwaites DI (Editors), Radiotherapy Physics in Practice, Oxford Medical Books, Oxford.

Baldwin RW, Byers VS, 1987, Monoclonal antibody targeting of cytotoxic agents for cancer therapy. In: Byers BS, Baldwin RW (Editors), Immunology of Malignant Disease, MTP Press, Lancaster.

Burns N, 1982, Nursing and Cancer, WB Saunders Co., Philadelphia.

Dillman JB, 1988, Toxicity of monoclonal antibodies in the treatment of cancer, Seminars in Oncology Nursing, **4**, 107-111.

Easson EC, 1985, General principles of radiotherapy. In: Easson EC, Pointon RCS (Editors), The Radiotherapy of Malignant Disease, Springer-Verlag, Berlin.

Flower MA, Chittenden SJ, 1993, Unsealed source therapy. In: Williams JR, Thwaites DI (Editors), Radiotherapy Physics in

Practice, Oxford Medical Books, Oxford.

Glicksman A, 1987, Radiobiologic basis of brachytherapy, Seminars in Oncology Nursing, **3**, 3-6.

Hall E, 1978, Radiobiology for the Radiologist (Second edition), Harper and Row, Philadelphia.

Hilderley LJ, Dow KH, 1991, Radiation oncology. In: Baird SB, McCorkle R, Grant M (Editors), Cancer Nursing: A Comprehensive Textbook, WB Saunders Co., Philadelphia.

Ionising Radiation Regulations, 1995, Schedule 1, Her Majesty's Stationery Office, London.

Morgan AC, Foon KA, 1986, Monoclonal antibody therapy of cancer: preclinical models and investigations in humans. In: Herberman KB (Editor), Cancer Immunology: Innovative Approaches in Therapy, Martinus Nijhoff Publishers, Boston.

Oldham RK, Smalley RV, 1983, Immunotherapy: the old and the new, Journal of Biological Response Modifiers, **2**, 1-37.

CHAPTER 13   EMERGENCY AND PALLIATIVE USE OF RADIOTHERAPY

Somewhere approaching 50% of all radiotherapy is given with palliative intent since it is an effective means of relieving severe or distressing symptoms and can markedly increase the quality of life even when cure is unlikely. The aim of palliative treatment is the relief of a symptom(s) thus improving comfort and providing support for affected patients. For example, the distress associated with compression of the superior vena cava or spinal cord can be relieved by radiotherapy of short duration and the local discomfort and discharge of an ulcerated lesion reduced (Easson and Pointon, 1985). This emphasis on improving distressing symptoms rather than aiming for cure means that the method of treatment is significantly different since the objectives are such that acute side-effects are not tolerated although the risk of long-term effects is not usually a major concern (Ch 4). Thus the treatment plan is carefully designed to ensure that the treatment itself is as unstressful as possible. The criteria of good palliative care can be summarised as follows:

1. The symptom must be sufficiently disturbing and persistent to justify an effort to relieve it.
2. The treatment required to relieve that symptom must be of short duration and make no additional demands on the patient.
3. The radiation dose required should be adequate to meet the desired objective without creating any side-effects.

(Easson and Pointon, 1985)

Treatment that fails to meet these criteria is bad palliative care since, clearly, treatment which creates further symptoms, or adds further distress, has failed to meet its desired objectives.

PAIN

The pain associated with malignant disease is often chronic and disabling and can totally disrupt the life of many sufferers. Early and aggressive treatment directed towards its relief is an essential part of care. When pain is due to local causes, such as bone metastases, radiotherapy can provide effective pain relief, and may also prevent pathological fractures of the affected area (Blitzer 1985). Indeed,

178

Blitzer (1985) has shown that up to 55% of all patients with bone metastasis experience significant and long-lasting pain relief which usually within days of the therapy, although its success is dependant on the radiosensitivity of the tumour. Systemic chemotherapy may be used in combination with radiotherapy when lesions are extensive. Other causes of pain, such as the extent or site of the tumour, may also be effectively relieved by radiation therapy.

PATHOLOGICAL FRACTURES

Pathological fractures commonly arise following the progressive bone destruction that may be associated with metastatic disease (e.g. lung, breast, prostate and lymphoma amongst others). Indeed, they affect about 8% of all patients with cancer (Faehnrich, 1983) most commonly involving the spine, ribs, long bones and sternum (Chernecky and Krech, 1991). Vertebral collapse is not uncommon and may cause pain, kyphosis, scoliosis and some degree of restrictive lung disease (Coleman, 1996). Internal fixation is the treatment of choice where this is possible, followed by radiotherapy. If the patient is not fit for surgery then radiotherapy and non-weight-bearing are indicated. However, although radiotherapy can provide effective pain relief, and may also prevent pathological fractures of affected areas (Blitzer 1985), it is less useful in treating pathological fractures once they have occurred. Untreated fractures rarely heal even though radiotherapy may achieve local control of the tumour itself (Coleman, 1986). Thus, once a fracture has occurred internal fixation is the only method of treatment that is likely to result in a return of function.

INCREASED INTRACRANIAL PRESSURE (see Ch 7)

Raised intracranial pressure is, classically, manifested by periodic frontal or bioccipital headaches, projectile vomiting and mental torpor accompanied by papilloedema. The patient may develop personality changes, is often unsteady and may be incontinent of urine and/or faeces. These effects require immediate treatment (Adams and Victor, 1985; Salcman and Kaplan, 1986) if coma and/or death are to be avoided. Other, more specific symptoms may occur depending on the site of the lesion.

In the past the only means by which raised intracranial pressure could be treated was through surgical intervention. Nowadays, although there are still patients who require surgical treatment, a variety of medical measures can preclude the need for surgery. The choice of treatment is determined largely by the severity of the condition as well as the physical status of the patient.

Treatment with corticosteroids, particularly dexamethasone, is often the method of choice when their effects reduce inflammation, prevent increased capillary permeability and promote diuresis (Ch 7).

However, in many cases, increased intracranial pressure results from either an intracranial tumour or metastatic tumour spread when radiotherapy is the primary method of treatment; radiation may also be helpful when the patient's condition precludes surgical intervention. This may be carried out using whole-head teletherapy or interstitial therapy.

SPINAL CORD COMPRESSION

This is a devastating complication of advanced malignancy primarily occurring in patients with metastatic disease. It can develop from metastatic tumours which infiltrate the epidural space and put pressure on the spinal cord and account for about 95% of its total incidence. Of these, solid tumours account for some 50% of all affected patients (Bruckman and Bloomer, 1978). Tumours of the lung, breast and prostate carry the highest risk accounting for 16%, 12% and 7% respectively. It may also be due to fracture dislocation of damaged vertebrae since such tumours often metastasise to the vertebral bodies (Coleman, 1996). It may also arise in myeloma while lymphoma and neuroblastoma may extend into the spinal cord (Cairncross and Posner, 1981).

Spinal cord compression is a serious condition and, unless prompt and effective emergency care is initiated, will cause permanent neurological damage. Damage to the spinal cord may result from compressive or invasive tumour growth and the severity depends in the location of the tumour.

Extradural involvement is the most common accompaniment to invasive growth which tends to invade the vertebral body and progress to the epidural space. This causes symptoms due to vertebral destruction, blockage of the cerebrospinal fluid and pressure on the spinal cord. Intradural metastasis is rare. Tumours are generally the result of primary spinal tumours, such as angioma or glioma, although they may reach the intradural space by haematogenous spread. Occasionally vertebral metastases will extend directly into the intradural space (Figure 13.1).

Figure 13.1   Spinal cord compression

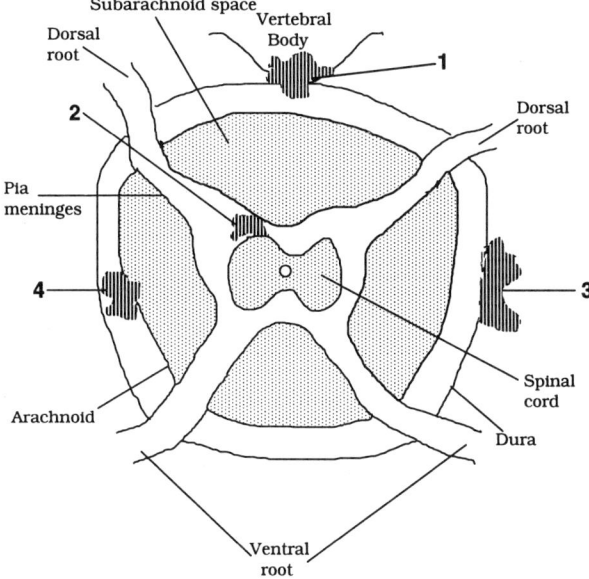

1. Bony metastases of a vertebra outside spinal column
2. Intramedullary tumour
3. Extradural tumour within spinal canal
4. Extramedullary tumour

Since the spinal cord carries both motor and sensory fibres, partial cord compression may result in unequal patterns of motor and sensory loss; total transection will result in paralysis below the level of transection. Compression also leads to oedema of the cord and ischaemia which mechanically distort/damage neural tissues (Dietz and Flaherty, 1992).

Typical history

Since more than 90% of affected patients have central back pain, which may or may not radiate, the history is typically one of progressive back pain that occurs for perhaps 6 months before diagnosis is confirmed. This is usually the presenting system although some patients will complain of weakness with or without numbness of the legs. There is usually a history of metastatic disease. This is described as the prodromal phase during which the pain may be exacerbated by lying down, coughing and moving and can often be alleviated by sitting upright. There may be an extended

181

period during which the pain is characterised by a diffuse or referred pain although, as the tumour increases in size causing chronic compression, the intensity, character and referral patterns may change; motor weakness may be present. Alternatively, severe and agonising pain may indicate vertebral collapse and be accompanied by paralysis that develops over several hours. At this stage, spinal tenderness and local kyphosis are likely.

The emergency, compressive phase follows. The resultant severity and impairment of neurological function are entirely dependent on the site of the tumour and the speed with which the diagnosis is made and treatment commenced.

Treatment

The importance of early recognition and diagnosis cannot be over-emphasised; early treatment is of equal importance. The objective of treatment is to relieve the compression as rapidly as possible so as to prevent further damage to the spinal cord. All patients should be started on high-dose corticosteroids to reduce oedema around the site of the compression until treatment decisions are made (Coleman, 1996). Although such therapy is valuable in acute control of this distressing condition, these drugs should be reduced as soon as possible to prevent steroid-related side-effects (Table 7.3).

The choice of treatment lies between surgery and radiotherapy and the decision is dependant on a variety of factors including the nature of the underlying disease and its prognosis, the patient's general condition and the severity of neurological damage. Surgical decompression is usually performed only on those patients who are reasonably fit and who have rapidly progressing neurological damage of recent onset (i.e. < 24hrs) (Coleman, 1996). All other patients are treated with radiotherapy commonly using doses of 3000-4000cGy over a 2-4 week period and dexamethasone to decrease inflammation, reduce pain and improve neurological function. This approach can restore some, or all, function depending on the severity of the compression. Radiation-induced side-effects are minimal and relate to the location of the treatment field on the spinal cord. Concurrent or subsequent chemotherapy may be given if the tumour is known to be chemosensitive.

Surgical decompression may, however, be indicated, for example when there is an inadequate response to the treatment outlined above or when there is a need for stabilisation of the spinal column.

Other indications for surgery include high cervical lesions that may cause respiratory distress, an uncertain diagnosis or prior radiotherapy in which spinal tolerance has been reached. In most cases surgery is followed by radiotherapy to destroy any remaining tumour cells.

SUPERIOR VENA CAVA SYNDROME (SVCS)

Compression of the superior vena cava (SVC) is a medical emergency which often responds to radiotherapy; this is the treatment of choice. Recognition, assessment and prompt action are essential since the SVC is the major vessel returning blood to the heart. Obstruction will result in an increase in venous pressure, dilation of superficial veins and will interfere with venous drainage.

Approximately 95% of all cases of SVC obstruction are due to malignancy when it results from compression by a tumour *per se* or from metastatic disease affecting the paratracheal or mediastinal lymph nodes which may create significant lymphadenopathy. Alternatively, the vessel walls may be infiltrated by the tumour causing the formation of a thrombus within the lumen. Thrombosis is also an increasingly common complication of the use of long-term central venous catheters frequently used in cancer patients and may cause SVC compression. Carcinoma of the bronchus is the most common underlying malignancy although breast cancer and lymphoma are other frequent causes (Carabell and Goodman, 1985; Coleman, 1996).

Typical history

Most commonly patients complain of dyspnoea accompanied by swelling of the face and neck and, occasionally, swelling of the trunk and upper extremities. Dysphagia, coughing and chest pain are also common and disturbances of the central nervous system, such as headache, visual disturbances and an altered state of consciousness, may also occur although these are rare. Symptoms are caused by the elevated venous pressure and congestion; their severity depends on the rapidity, degree and location of the obstruction. Rapidly developing SVCS may be fatal while gradual onset may allow a collateral circulation to develop which will shunt enough blood to minimise the complications (Simpson et al, 1981).

Clinically the patient will present with distension of the thoracic and neck veins, facial oedema and a rapid respiratory rate associated with cyanosis and, on occasions, oedema of the upper extremities. Disruption of the cervical nerve supply may cause vocal cord paralysis so that the patient becomes hoarse and finds difficulty in talking. In severe cases, airway obstruction can develop rapidly leading to respiratory arrest.

Diagnosis is confirmed by X-ray when significant findings include evidence of a right, superior mediastinal mass, paratracheal or mediastinal lymphadenopathy and right-sided effusion. At times, SVC obstruction will occur before the histology of the lesion has been established; bronchoscopy and/or biopsy of the lesion will be performed. However, when the patient is in acute distress, treatment may be undertaken even in the absence of a confirmed diagnosis. A diagnostic work-up is then carried out when the patient's condition has improved.

Treatment

Immediate care includes oxygen therapy and nursing the patient in an upright position. High-dose corticosteroids are given, usually dexamethasone at a dose of 12-16mg/day (Coleman, 1996). The prime goal of treatment is to relieve the obstruction and restore venous drainage by reducing the size of the tumour. This is most effectively achieved using radiotherapy which may be administered even in the absence of a tissue diagnosis. This usually results in rapid symptomatic relief within the first few days of treatment.

High-dose radiotherapy will result in rapid shrinking of the tumour. The precise dose and fractionation depend on the nature of the underlying tumour and are, typically, in the range of 20-30Gy over 5-10 daily fractions. This may be followed by smaller daily fractions until the desired dose, usually 300-350Gy is reached (Perez et al, 1985). In SVCS that is developing more slowly, a low-dose schedule may be followed when a constant daily dose of 150-200cGy is given throughout treatment. This will provide symptomatic relief for the majority of patients, usually within 3-7 days, particularly when appropriate supportive care is given. Oxygen therapy will help to relieve dyspnoea and analgesia and/or tranquillisers to decrease chest pain and anxiety. When oedema is present diuretics may provide temporary relief.

Although concurrent chemotherapy may be given in those with lymphoma or small-cell lung cancer, surgery is of only limited benefit in the treatment of SVCS and, in addition, carries a high morbidity rate. As a result it is rarely used as a method of treatment. Chemotherapy is occasionally used instead of radiotherapy in those tumours that are known to be chemosensitive. In this case the response is considerably less rapid.

CARDIAC TAMPONADE

Cardiac tamponade is an uncommon complication of malignancy. It is a life-threatening condition which results in an increase in intra-pericardial pressure. It may be due to an accumulation of fluid (pericardial effusion) or to constriction due to thickening (fibrosis). This, in turn, causes cardiac compression and decreased ventricular (diastolic) filling so that both the stroke volume and the cardiac output are decreased thus impairing systemic perfusion. At the same time distension of the pericardium will compress the lungs and bronchi resulting in dyspnoea and orthopnoea.

The condition may, or may not, be accompanied by chest pain but is characterised by distension of the jugular veins, muffled heart sounds, cyanosis, oedema, râles, an irregular pulse of decreased pressure, decreased systolic blood pressure and raised central venous pressure all of which, ultimately, lead to cardiac failure and shock and, if untreated, to death. Pain, when present, varies in intensity ranging from mild to severe over the precordial or sub-sternal area and may radiate to the shoulder and down the left arm; it may be aggravated by swallowing, coughing and lying flat and relieved by sitting up and leaning forward. Alternatively pain may be dull, diffuse and oppressive.

Cardiac tamponade may arise from a primary tumour of the heart that may, rarely, involve the pericardium (Mauch and Ullman, 1985) although it is more commonly due to secondary involvement by tumours of the lung or breast, to lymphoma or leukaemia, or to melanoma. It may also be due to previous radiation therapy; a total dose in the range of 4000-6000cGy delivered to a large portion of the heart, may result in radiation pericarditis and pericardial thickening (Appelfeld et al, 1981). Cardiac tamponade may be caused by either an abnormal accumulation of fluid in the pericardial space or, less commonly, by constrictive fibrosis of the pericardial space. As the effusion increases in size so the function of the right ventricle progressively declines resulting in the symptoms of right heart failure. Affected patients will be anxious and apprehensive.

Clearly an affected patient is acutely ill and requires emergency treatment. Bed rest is initiated and vital signs and cardiac function are monitored. Oxygen therapy, analgesics and/or sedatives are given as required and the patient is prepared for emergency treatment. The immediate goal of therapy is to achieve haemodynamic stability and to remove the pericardial effusion; this will provide immediate relief. The most appropriate method of achieving this is by inserting a catheter into the pericardial space, under ultrasound guidance, and allowing the fluid to drain over 24-48 hours (Coleman, 1996). Corticosteroids may help to reduce inflammation.

Radiotherapy was once the treatment of choice, provided, of course, that the condition was not due to radiation pericarditis. However, although this approach is no longer recommended (Coleman, 1996), it is still occasionally employed; a total dose of 2-300Gy is usually administered. This is adequate to relieve the symptoms but carries the risk of further damage to both the pericardium and myocardium.

When neither of these treatments are possible, a surgical opening (pericardial window) may be made to drain fluid to the pleural space and provide prolonged palliation. Advances in intracavity therapy have meant that recurrent pericardial effusions can now be treated by means of intrapericardial instillation of cytotoxic agents (e.g. cisplatin) (Markman and Howell, 1985).

Other malignant effusions (e.g. pleural effusion) can also cause distressing symptoms such as chest pain, dyspnoea, cough, tiredness and dysphagia and can, at times, be successfully treated by either teletherapy or brachytherapy provided that radiation-induced damage was not the initiating cause. Finally, radiotherapy can be used to suppress gross haemorrhage when a decrease or complete cessation of bleeding can be achieved (Rotman, 1976).

REFERENCES

Adams RD, Victor M, 1985, Principles of Neurology (Third edition), McGraw-Hill, New York.

Appelfeld MM, Cole JF, Pollock SH et al, 1981, The late appearance of chronic pericardial disease in patients treated by radiotherapy for Hodgkin's disease, Annals of Internal Medicine, **94**, 338-341.

Blitzer PH, 1985, Reanalysis of the RTOB study of the palliation of symptomatic osseous metastases, Cancer, **55**, 1468-1472.

Bruckman JE, Bloomer WD, 1978, Management of spinal cord

compression, Seminars in Oncology, **5**, 135-140.

Cairncross JG, Posner JB, 1981, Neurological complications of systemic cancer. In: Yarbro JW, Bornstein RS (Editors), Oncologic Emergencies, Grune and Stratton, New York.

Carabell SC, Goodman RL, 1985, Oncological emergencies: superior vena cava syndrome, In: DeVita VT, Hellman S, Rosenberg SA (Editors), Cancer Principles and Practice of Oncology, JB Lippincott, Philadelphia.

Chernecky C, Krech RL, Complications of Advanced disease. In: Baird SB, McCorkle R, Grant M (Editors), Cancer Nursing: A Comprehensive Textbook, WB Saunders Co., Philadelphia.

Coleman RE, 1996, Oncological emergencies. In: Hancock B (Editor) Cancer Care in the Community, Radcliffe Medical Press Ltd., Oxford.

Dietz KA, Flaherty AM, 1992 Oncological Emergencies. In: Groenwald SL, Frogge MH, Goodman M, Yarbro CH (Editors), Manifestations of Cancer and Cancer Treatments. Part V from Cancer Nursing: Principles and Practice (Second edition), Jones and Bartlett Publishers, Boston.

Easson EC, Pointon RCS, 1985, The Radiotherapy of Malignant Disease, Springer-Verlag, New York.

Faehnrich J, 1983, When pathologic fractures threaten, RN, **46**(11), 34-37.

Markman M, Howell SB, 1985, Intrapericardial instillation of cis-platin in a patient with a large malignant effusion, Cancer Drug Delivery, **2**, 49-52.

Mauch PM, Ullman JE, 1985, Treatment of malignant pericardial effusions. In: DeVita VT, Hellman S, Rosenberg SA (Editors), Cancer Principles and Practice of Oncology, JB Lippincott, Philadelphia.

Perez C, Presant C, Van Amburg A, 1985, Management of superior vena cava syndrome, Seminars in Oncology, **5**, 123-134.

Rotman M, 1976, Supportive and palliative radiation therapy, Ca: A Cancer Journal for Clinicians, **26**, 293-298.

Salcman M, Kaplan RS, 1986, Intracranial tumours in adults. In: Moosa AR, Robson MC, Schimpff SC (Editors), Comprehensive Textbook of Oncology, Williams and Wilkins, Baltimore.

Simpson JR, Perez CA, Presant CA et al, 1981, Superior vena cava syndrome, In: Yarbro JW, Bornstein RS (Editors), Oncology Emergencies, Grune and Stratton, New York.

CHAPTER 14   NUTRITIONAL CARE OF THE PATIENT UNDERGOING RADIOTHERAPY

The nutritional condition of a cancer patient undergoing radiotherapy is affected by both the disease and the treatment. Thus nutritional care cannot be discussed without first considering the nutritional effects of cancer itself (see Holmes and Dickerson, 1988). The effects of radiotherapy may exacerbate the decline in nutritional status.

NUTRITIONAL EFFECTS OF MALIGNANCY

Malnutrition affects some 40% of those hospitalised for treatment of cancer (Landel et al, 1985) and is associated with varying degrees of weight loss, a poor prognosis, a reduced response to therapy, prolonged or enhanced morbidity of therapeutic side-effects and a reduced quality of life. Weight loss may arise even before the diagnosis is made or confirmed and is often one of the most disabling aspects of the disease leading to distressing and potentially life-threatening symptoms (such as secondary infection). It occurs at different stages in the disease and does not directly correlate with the histological type or site of the tumour, the extent of metastasis, duration of disease or with food intake. Such weight loss leads to marked decreases in both body fat and muscle mass leading to wasting and physical weakness and provoking anxiety for patients and carers. This condition is known as cancer cachexia, the term 'cachexia' being derived from the Greek 'kaxos' and 'hexis' meaning poor condition.

A number of symptoms characterise cachexia including anorexia, early satiety, marked weight loss, muscle weakness, anaemia and oedema that accompany the symptoms of the primary disease. Such symptoms result from the cumulative effects of various factors including alterations in energy requirements and disturbances of carbohydrate, protein and fat metabolism. These combine with the primary symptoms further exacerbating nutritional decline. For example, malabsorption may potentiate nutrient deficiency while pain, depression, fatigue, anxiety, and other symptoms, may potentiate anorexia; treatment-induced effects may exacerbate such symptoms still further.

In view of the significant morbidity and mortality associated with cachexia considerable research has been devoted to attempts to identify ways of overcoming its undesirable effects. Better understanding and reversal of its deleterious effects would not only improve well-being but also the life expectancy of many patients (Gelin and Lundholm, 1992). Yet malnutrition can often be avoided (Shils, 1977) and, as cancer is a chronic disease, this emphasises the need for nutritional support to be initiated early in the disease process; it is easier to prevent malnutrition than it is to rehabilitate the already malnourished. The short-term benefits of nutritional care may markedly improve both well-being and quality of life (Torosian et al, 1983; Holmes and Dickerson, 1991).

PATHOPHYSIOLOGY OF MALNUTRITION
The development of malnutrition involves many complex factors (Table 14.1) and both cancer itself and its treatment may contribute to its occurrence. Its extent is also influenced by the location of the tumour; malnutrition is more common with tumours at specific sites, such as the head and neck, gastrointestinal tract, central nervous system and lung as well as aggressive lymphomas (Ollenschlager et al, 1988). However, no patient and no tumour are excluded.

Table 14.1   Causes of malnutrition in the cancer patient.

Metabolic disorders - alterations in the metabolism of fat, protein, carbohydrate, vitamins, minerals and electrolytes
Anorexia
Taste aberrations
Dysphagia
Malabsorption
Food aversion
Early satiety
Emotional/psychological consequences of disease and treatment
Treatment-induced side-effects

Protein-energy malnutrition (PEM) is the most common form of malnutrition and develops when dietary protein and energy intake are insufficient to meet individual needs. An inadequate intake leads to mobilisation of body nutrient stores to meet the nutrient demand so that fat and protein are catabolised to provide energy. This results in a loss of both subcutaneous fat and muscle mass; visceral proteins, such as serum albumin and transferrin, are also depleted. However, in cancer, PEM reflects not only a reduced consumption but also an increased demand for nutrients. Malignant tumours may act as 'parasites' drawing nutrients from the host. When dietary intake does not meet the nutrient demands of both host and tumour, body stores are catabolised and weight falls. Yet Morrison (1976), argued that 'normal' individuals increase their intake when energy requirements are increased. Clearly, this does not occur in cancer and food intake does not keep pace with nutrient needs. Indeed, some patients fail even to maintain their current weight, despite intakes of 3-4000kcal/day (Heber et al, 1985). Thus, in the absence of obvious causative factors, such as co-existent endocrine disorders or sepsis, it seems that malignancy *per se* induces profound nutritional abnormalities. These are manifested by significant metabolic changes (Table 14.2) which result in an increased demand for energy and lead to depletion of body protein stores (from muscle) and fat (from subcutaneous tissue). Although anorexia may contribute to body tissue depletion it is quite clear that inadequate food consumption alone cannot account for these effects; other factors must also contribute to their development.

Table 14.2   **Examples of the metabolic changes which may be associated with cancer**

Metabolic change	Effect	Manifestations
↑ energy expenditure	↑ energy demand ↑ basal metabolic rate ↑ protein catabolism	Weight loss Loss of subcutaneous fat Loss of body protein Muscle weakness
Alterations in glucose metabolism	Impaired glucose tolerance ↑ anaerobic glycolysis ↑ gluconeogenesis ↓ sensitivity to insulin ↓ energy production	Hyperglycaemia Protein depletion leading to muscle weakness
↓ protein synthesis		Protein depletion leading to muscle weakness Immunodepression
↑ fat catabolism		Loss of subcutaneous fat Decrease in total body fat Weight loss

Possible mechanisms of metabolic change

Research indicates that some tumours produce substances that induce metabolic derangements and Beutler and Cerami (1986) have

Nutritional care of the patient undergoing radiotherapy

suggested that the immune system is significant in mediating such effects. Cachectin [tumour necrosis factor (TNF)], for example, when given to animals, induces anorexia and weight loss that are consistent with human cachexia; it has also been implicated in the cachexia of chronic disease (Kawakami and Cerami, 1981). Thus it seems that cachectin-induced catabolism may account for at least some of the physical wasting accompanying malignancy (Torti et al, 1985). It may be that cachectin (TNF) 'orchestrates' at least some of the complex metabolic changes contributing to the development of cachexia (Beutler and Cerami, 1986).

In addition, progressive malignancy is known to be accompanied by an acute phase response (Cooper and Stone, 1979) similar to that evoked by other tissue injuries (e.g. inflammation or sepsis) which can cause cachexia if prolonged and untreated (Gelin and Lundholm, 1992). The similarity in physiological responses suggests involvement of common mediator(s) (e.g. TNF). Similarly, interleukin-1 (IL-1) and interleukin-6 (IL-6), often used in biological therapy, induce cachexia in experimental animals and, like TNF, provoke an acute phase response in the liver (Selby et al, 1987). Both TNF and IL-1 exert autocrine and paracrine actions (Figure 14.1) which, in turn, stimulate IL-6 release; IL-6 potentiates anorexia (Busbridge et al, 1989). It is, therefore, possible that local production of both TNF and IL-1 contributes to the development of cachexia in some patients; it is, however, unlikely to be its major cause (Fearon, 1992).

Figure 14.1   The action of cytokines

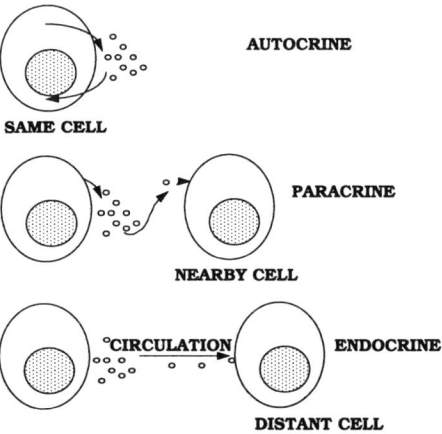

191

Fluid and electrolyte disturbances

Fluid and electrolyte disturbances are common systemic symptoms and, in advanced cancer, both intra- and extracellular water are increased thus masking body tissue loss so that, as disease progresses, the value of body weight as an indicator of nutritional depletion declines.

Hyponatraemia and hypercalcaemia are the most common electrolyte disturbances seen. Indeed malignancy is the most common cause of hypercalcaemia in hospital patients. Complications of both the disease and its treatment may cause other electrolyte abnormalities and acid-base imbalance.

Weight loss and hypercatabolism can stimulate sodium and potassium loss although serum levels remain in the normal range. Hypocalcaemia may arise in the presence of hypoalbuminaemia. Serum electrolytes must, therefore, be closely monitored.

Impaired food intake

Food intake may be impaired by many factors (Table 14.1). The location of a tumour may affect ingestion, digestion or absorption and malignancy anywhere in the body may cause malabsorption through secondary intestinal changes (Wangel and Deller, 1966).

Anorexia (Ch 6) commonly compounds cancer-associated weight loss; various factors contribute to its development. For example, metabolic effects may generate spurious signals that are interpreted centrally as indicators of satiety (Mattes et al, 1987) so that the patient feels full whether or not he has eaten adequate amounts.

Serotonin, and other neurotransmitters, have been the focus of most research in this area. For example, Krause et al (1979a; 1979b) have shown that cerebral serotonin levels correlate closely with the onset of anorexia. This, together with suggestions that serotonin plays a role in generating satiety (e.g. Lehr and Goldman, 1973; Kruk, 1976), led to the hypothesis that serotonin may be linked to the development of anorexia; others, however (e.g. von Meyendfeldt et al, 1980), have shown that inhibiting serotonin synthesis does not eliminate anorexia suggesting that other mechanisms are also involved.

Although such work offers the possibility of clinical intervention to control anorexia, further work is required.

Behavioural and symptomatic factors: Although metabolic changes are clearly important in the development of malnutrition, the contribution of behavioural and symptomatic factors cannot be over-looked. For example, emotional responses may adversely affect appetite and there are times in the disease trajectory when patients are particularly vulnerable to emotional distress.

Considerable stress is experienced before the diagnosis is confirmed. Confirmation may promote further emotional trauma; a weight loss of 5-10lbs is not unusual during this period, primarily due to psychological or emotional factors rather than the disease itself (Holland et al, 1977).

Previous attitudes and beliefs about cancer and its treatment may combine with continued fear of recurrence, appearance of new symptoms (whether or not they are disease-related) and anxiety related to cancer treatments, contributing to the causation of anorexia (Schmale, 1979). Thus anorexia may be experienced as an emotional response throughout the course of the disease.

Similarly, depression may accompany continued progression of the disease and could provide a psychological basis for anorexia. This would, therefore, be expected to improve with antidepressive therapy. However, anorexia is generally unresponsive to tricyclic drug therapy (Wesdorp et al, 1983) and, since Plumb et al (1976) showed that, although physical symptoms are common, non-physical signs of depression (e.g. feelings of worthlessness, guilt, suicidal tendencies) are not significant, it can be suggested that depression does not contribute significantly to its aetiology. In any case, Holland et al (1977) claim that symptoms suggestive of depression reflect the physical rather than the psychological condition.

Physical discomfort: Any type of physical discomfort may depress food intake; control of distressing symptoms is essential. Such discomfort may include the stomatitis, xerostomia, pain, nausea and vomiting or diarrhoea caused by radiotherapy.

Taste changes. Alterations in appetite and anorexia may both be attributable to taste changes which, together with an altered sense of smell (anosmia), may lead to disinterest in food. Positive taste experiences are important in triggering the physiological responses contributing to food ingestion and digestion. For example, the volume of salivary and gastric secretions depends, in part, on individual taste experiences. Thus, when taste changes are present, the taste stimulus may be inadequate to stimulate appropriate physiological reactions thus contributing to malnutrition and weight loss.

Food Aversion: Learned food aversion (Ch 6) is not uncommon and may play a major role in decreasing food consumption (e.g. Bernstein and Bernstein, 1981; Leathwood et al, 1986).

Psychosocial factors influencing nutritional status

As has been shown, both emotional and behavioural factors associated with diagnosis and treatment may contribute to malnutrition by reducing food intake. That anxiety occurs cannot be doubted. For example, Peck and Boland (1977) focused on patients' attitudes towards radiotherapy showing that 60% experienced significant levels of anxiety before treatment; this rose to 80% following completion of therapy. Such effects could clearly decrease the appetite.

Hospital-related factors

Hospitalisation may, itself, adversely affect eating patterns due to the timing of meals and/or the types of food available since this may disrupt the patient's normal routine; cultural factors may influence the type(s) of food that patients are able or willing to eat. Eating behaviour is influenced by a wide variety of social, cultural, psychological and physiological factors (Novin and van der Weele, 1977; Holmes, 1987) all of which may be disrupted by cancer and its treatment, compounding the nutritional problems to which affected patients are exposed.

Eating is normally a social event but, in hospitals, there are rarely common eating places and patients may be left to eat in isolation, in bed or at the bed side, reducing social interaction. Food is often served in large, impersonal portions that seem to take no note of individual needs or requests. It is difficult to allow for individual likes and dislikes but, in cancer, a flexible and individual approach is essential if food intake and, therefore, nutritional status is to be maintained.

Certain procedures can potentiate nutritional decline. For example, although investigations are essential in hospital care they may be associated with unnecessarily prolonged starvation; this may be extended by pre- and post-operative fasting. Missing meals is sometimes unavoidable but alternative provision should be made to ensure that food intake is maintained. However, administrative changes have made this more difficult (Garrow, 1994). Catering services may be provided on tightly controlled contracts; additional meals, or even snacks, often require dietetic referral while hygiene regulations prohibit preparation or storage of food in ward kitchens. Thus those patients fasted overnight for diagnostic tests, and absent from the ward at lunch, may wait as long as 24hrs between meals. It is little wonder that already malnourished patients often lose more weight in hospital (Garrow, 1994). This may be exacerbated when necessary assistance or feeding aids are not available to patients in need. The importance of attempting to overcome such difficulties cannot be over-emphasised.

NUTRITIONAL MANAGEMENT OF THE RADIOTHERAPY PATIENT

The preceding discussion shows that patients undergoing radiotherapy may have a compromised nutritional status before treatment begins and, as we have seen, many of its side-effects may have nutritional consequences exacerbating malnutrition. In addition, many may have received prior therapy which may have long-lasting nutritional consequences (Table 14.3).

This means that nutritional care is an essential part of the total care of the patient undergoing radiotherapy to help them to cope and to enhance both the therapeutic response and the quality of life. It is clear that appetite and the ability to eat are important factors in determining the quality of life (Padilla, 1986).

Nutritional assessment

Although prevention of malnutrition must be the primary aim, nutritional care is often considered only after the patient is severely depleted. The initial care plan for all radiotherapy patients should include nutritional assessment both to determine the risk of nutritional depletion and to provide background data against which the severity of future changes can be assessed. Periodic follow-up assessment should be carried out at least once a month even after nutritional support has been instigated. This enables care to be dynamic and responsive to the patient's changing needs. The overall goals of such care are:

1. To prevent or correct nutritional deficiencies.
2. To prevent or minimise weight loss.

Nutritional assessment is the essential first step in developing a care plan and is important for all patients whether in hospital or the community. It describes the process through which the nutritional condition is established and represents the degree to which individual needs for nutrients are met by the nutrient consumption.

195

Table 14.3   Some treatment-induced nutritional effects

Surgery	Oropharyngeal	Chewing/swallowing difficulties
		Dependence on enteral (tube)
		feeding
	Oesophagectomy	Gastric stasis
		Hypochorhydria
		Diarrhoea/steatorrhoea
	Gastrectomy	Achlorhydria and lack of intrinsic
		factor → vitamin B_{12} malabsorption
		Hypoglycaemia
		Dumping syndrome
		General malabsorption
	Intestinal: jejunal	Malabsorption
	ileum	Vitamin B_{12} deficiency
		Bile salt deficiency
		Diarrhoea
	massive	Severe malabsorption
		Acidosis
	Ileostomy/colostomy	Fluid/electrolyte imbalance
Radiotherapy	General	Radiation syndrome
		Anorexia
	Head and neck	Altered taste sensation
		Xerostomia
		Damage to, or loss of, teeth
		Mucositis
	Lower neck or	Oeophagitis, pharyngitis
	mediastinum	Dysphagia
		Fibrosis, oesophageal stenosis or
		stricture
	Abdomen/pelvis	Acute/chronic bowel damage
		Diarrhoea
		Malabsorption
		Intestinal fistulae, fibrosis or
		stenosis
Chemotherapy		Anorexia
		Nausea and vomiting
		Diarrhoea/constipation
		Stomatitis/mucositis
		Intestinal ulceration
		Malabsorption
	Corticosteroids	Fluid and electrolyte
		disturbances
		Nitrogen and calcium losses
		Hyperglycaemia

If carried out effectively nutritional assessment helps to:
- Identify existing/potential problems
- Identify the cause of current problems
- Provide baseline data for subsequent assessment
- Determine the response to nutritional intervention.

Clinical observation, anthropometric techniques, biochemical analyses and dietary evaluation are the general methods of nutritional assessment although this should also include socio-economic and pyschosocial factors. Much of this information should be provided through a thorough nursing assessment. Discussion with family and friends may provide valuable additional information.

Current drug therapy should also be identified, including not only antineoplastic therapy but also vitamins and other 'over-the-counter' medicines and 'recreational' drugs (Holmes, 1986). Additional health problems, such as diabetes mellitus or renal disease, must be recognised since these may, themselves, affect nutrition.

Clinical examination includes observation of the general condition and, with a complete physical examination, reflects overall nutritional status. Although the physical signs and symptoms of malnutrition may not be evident until the condition is advanced, weight loss, for example, may be visible to the naked eye.

Particular attention should be paid to examining the skin, hair, mouth, teeth and general skin and muscle tone since these may provide evidence of nutritional deficiency. Common signs indicating malnutrition include: dry, flaky skin, dull or sunken eyes, oral lesions, muscle wasting or oedema; sparse or thin hair may also be evident. Psychosocial factors that should be considered include levels of anxiety, fear or depression all of which may potentiate anorexia.

Anthropometric data (Table 14.4) are central to any physical examination. These represent physical measurements reflecting nutritional status. Some, such as height, indicate past or chronic nutritional status whilst others (e.g. skinfold thickness and midarm circumference) reflect the current nutritional condition and are used to assess skeletal energy reserves. Such data is most useful when obtained over a period of time so that the initial assessment provides an important baseline for subsequent assessment.

The degree of energy depletion is determined by the height:weight index, triceps skinfold thickness (TSF) and the midarm circumference (MAC). Weight and height are the most common measures of nutritional status but, because their nutritional status is often not

Table 14.4   Anthropometric measurements in nutritional assessment

	Purpose	Technique
Body weight	Provides basis for other anthropometric measures. Sum of all body constituents - repeated measures will indicate changes.	Use same scale, clothing and time of day. Empty bladder and bowel before weighing.
Height	Represents past (chronic) nutritional status. Used with weight to calculate ideal body weight.	See text.
Ideal body weight (IBW)	Once calculated provides an indication of nutritional status. A current weight 70-80% IBW indicates moderate malnutrition; <70% IBW = severe malnutrition.	Calculated from height and weight using standard tables.
Usual body weight (UBW)	Once usual body weight has been established it becomes possible to calculate the percentage weight change. Useful indicator of nutritional change.	$$\% \text{ UBW} = \frac{\text{Current weight (kg)}}{\text{UBW (kg)}} \times 100$$ % weight change $$= \frac{\text{UBW (kg) - current weight (kg)}}{\text{UBW (kg)}} \times 100$$
Midarm circumference (MAC)	Reflects body protein and fat content.	Measure circumference of upper arm at mid-point between acromial process of scapula and olecranon process of ulna using a non-stretchable tape measure.
Triceps skinfold thickness (TSF)	Estimates subcutaneous fat and energy reserves.	Measure at same point as MAC using callipers. Take average of 3 readings. Ensure skin and fat lifted clear of underlying tissue prior to measurement.
Midarm muscle circumference (MAMC)	Provides further evidence with regard to body energy and protein reserves.	Estimated indirectly from MAC and TSF. MAMC = MAC (cm) - (3.142 x TSF
Arm muscle area (AMA)	Provides further evidence with regard to body energy and protein reserves.	$$\text{AMA (cm}^2) = \frac{(\text{MAMC - 3.142 x TSF})}{4 \times 3.142}$$ $$\text{AMA (cm}^2) = \frac{(\text{MAMC - 3.142 x TSF})}{4 \times 3.142}$$

[**Note:** These measurements provide only an approximate guide to changes in energy reserves. They are of most value when used to monitor patients over a period of time].

recognised, they are often measured sloppily and inconsistently. Since weight loss is associated with increased morbidity and mortality in cancer patients the importance of accuracy in measurement cannot be over-emphasised. For example, Johnston et al (1980) demonstrated that the oral pain, dysguesia, xerostomia and dysphagia associated with radiotherapy of the head and neck were both more severe and longer lasting in those with weight loss.

If weight is to be obtained accurately the patient should be weighed in the morning prior to breakfast and with an empty bladder. The same scales should be used, and clothes should be worn, each time the patient is weighed.

Height should be measured as described below:

1. The patient should be barefoot or wearing only socks or stockings.
2. His feet should be together with heels against the wall or measuring board.
3. He should be standing erect, not slumped or stretching, and looking straight ahead.
4. A horizontal bar is then lowered to rest flat against the top of the head.
5. Height is read to the nearest 0.5 cm.

To determine whether weight is appropriate for height (IBW) the weight is compared with standard tables. However, such figures can be misleading if they are used to determine whether an individual is at some 'desirable' weight (Durnin and Fidanza, 1985) since the concept of 'ideal body weight' is derived from life assurance tables. Although these relate weight and height to mortality they have limitations since the information is derived from a restricted, and possibly unrepresentative, sample of applicants for life assurance. It is also important to realise that, in cancer patients, the recorded body weight may be distorted by the presence of oedema or ascites as well as tumour mass.

Nonetheless, when current weight is compared with the usual body weight (prior to the diagnosis of cancer), this can provide a guide to the patient's weight change; weight loss is *always* significant. It is also important to remember that, although the current weight may be appropriate for height, this may still be significantly below the patient's usual weight. Estimating percentage weight change thus provides a more sensitive indicator of tissue gain or loss.

Triceps skinfold thickness (TSF) is a measurement of sub-cutaneous fat and, once measured, is compared with the reference standard tables (see Goodinson, 1987a). Because the amount of fat located in the subcutaneous tissues varies with age and sex it is important that tables used to evaluate skinfold measurements are age and sex specific.

Midarm circumference (MAC) provides a sensitive indicator of lean body mass and, therefore, of skeletal protein reserves. When MAC is combined with TSF it becomes possible to obtain an even better assessment of energy and protein nutriture, through indirect determination of the arm muscle and fat area. The arm muscle area provides a good indication of the lean body mass and, therefore, skeletal protein reserves, which is particularly valuable in assessing the patient who is likely to be protein-energy malnourished (such as the cancer patient) (see Wright and Heymsfield, 1985; Gibson, 1990). Since changes in both fat and protein mass provide good indicators of nutritional change they should be used at the initial assessment and serially to evaluate the nutritional changes resulting from cancer and its treatment.

Biochemical analyses provide important nutritional information and, as the most specific of all assessment techniques, can detect covert nutritional deficiencies. For example, serum albumin and transferrin are indicative of visceral protein levels; serum transferrin also reflects body protein synthesis. Serum albumin can also be used to identify vulnerable patients since hypoalbuminaemia is associated with an increased incidence of complications after cancer therapies (e.g. Kokal, 1985).

Immunocompetence is another important indicator that is significantly reduced by malnutrition. Cell-mediated immunity is particularly vulnerable to the effects of malnutrition. The total lymphocyte count reflects immunocompetence as well as visceral protein stores and is decreased in those with protein-energy malnutrition. Skin sensitivity tests to recall antigens can be used to reflect T-cell-mediated immunity.

When cell-mediated immunity is impaired, the response to antigens to which individuals have previously been exposed is diminished; alternatively there may be a complete lack of response (anergy). Daly et al (1979) have shown that those who are anergic have, on average, lost 20kg more than those individuals with a functioning immune system.

However, concurrent disease and/or therapy may also cause immunosuppression thus limiting the value of these techniques in affected patients. Indeed, since metabolic disturbances are common, biochemical changes may reflect the presence of malignancy itself rather than nutritional abnormalities.

Nonetheless, when taken in conjunction with other measures of nutritional status, biochemical tests may be useful. An excellent discussion of the biochemical assessment of nutritional status is to be found in Goodinson (1987b).

Dietary evaluation. This may include both assessment of actual food and drink consumption and a history of prior intake and usual dietary habits.

However, although a dietary history (see later discussion) contributes valuable information, it is a difficult and often frustrating aspect of nutritional assessment since it is difficult to record a person's food intake without influencing eating patterns although the extent of the change depends on how well they understand the need for such measures and to what degree they are influenced by what they think the nurse or dietician wants to know. An awareness of this possibility is essential in assessing the data obtained.

The most common methods of assessing food consumption are dietary recall and direct observation (Table 14.5).

Standard food tables can be used to establish the actual nutrient consumption. Alternatively the food group method can be used to provide a crude measure of nutrient consumption (see Table 14.6); it will, however, enable detection of gross deficiencies of protein, iron, calcium and some vitamins although this can be more difficult when the diet comprises many mixed or unusual foods that cannot be easily classified.

It must, however, be recognised that the simple act of measuring food intake may significantly affect the amount and type of food consumed and the nutrient composition may be altered by the method of preparation and storage after cooking.

As a result, an accurate assessment of nutritional status relies on a combination of the methods discussed since it is neither possible nor accurate to judge the adequacy of the diet by looking at the intake alone. Serum and tissue levels of nutrients must also be evaluated and a thorough physical examination undertaken to assess the clinical evidence of a deficiency state.

Table 14.5   Recording of dietary intake

Method		Comment
24 hour recall	Interview/questionnaire designed to establish everything eaten in previous 24hrs and to obtain an estimate of the quantity.	Contains inherent sources of error because it is difficult to recall accurately everything that has been eaten; previous day's intake may not be typical; individual may not be telling the truth.
Food frequency questionnaire	Provides information on frequency of consumption of individual foods (e.g. how often it is eaten per day, week or month).	Can validate 24hr recall and clarify food consumption. May be selective looking at only those areas believed to be deficient.
Food diary	Patient records everything he eats/drinks over a defined period, usually 3-4 days. Often includes both week days and weekends.	Requires more time, understanding and motivation from the patient but, if recorded immediately after eating, provides accurate data. Problems include non-compliance, inaccuracy in recording or atypical intake on recording days.
Direct observation	Enables precise recording of food presented and consumed especially if food and waste are weighed. Should be as unobtrusive as possible and is most easily achieved when patient's meals are provided for him.	The most time-consuming, expensive and difficult method of obtaining dietary data. When weighed intakes are required can lead to difficulties with patient compliance.

A *dietary history* allows information regarding usual dietary habits to be obtained and should form a standard part of the nursing assessment of every cancer patient. This can help to:

- Establish whether the diet is sufficient
- Determine food likes, dislikes and preferences
- Evaluate current and previous eating patterns
- Provide information about social and environmental factors influencing the ability to purchase, obtain or prepare food
- Allow identification of factors inhibiting food consumption (e.g. chewing/swallowing difficulties, anorexia, nausea, and vomiting, oral discomfort)
- Identify concurrent illness (e.g. diabetes or renal disease)

Nutritional care of the patient undergoing radiotherapy

- Identify any dietary change occurring as a result of disease or treatment.

In obtaining such a history, discussion with family and friends may provide further useful information. A dietary history thus helps both to identify areas of difficulty for specific patients and to develop a nutritional care plan based on individual likes and dislikes, preferences and habits thus helping to increase the likelihood of compliance with any dietary regime.

Table 14.6   The basic food groups

	Number of servings per day	What is a serving?
Meat group	2 or more	2-3 oz lean, cooked meat, poultry or fish 1 egg 4 oz cooked, dried beans, peas or legumes 4 tbspns peanut butter
Milk group (adults)	2 or more	8 oz milk - whole, skimmed, buttermilk or evaporated milk 1.5 oz Cheddar-type cheese 8 oz cottage cheese 6 oz yoghurt 6 oz ice cream
Vegetable and fruit group	4 or more	6 oz vegetable 1 apple, banana, potato ½ medium grapefruit or melon
	plus 1 or 2 (vitamin C)	Grapefruit, orange, orange juice Brussels sprouts Green peppers Melon/lemon Cabbage, cress, spinach, cauliflower Potatoes, sweet potatoes, yams Tomatoes
	1 (at least every other day - vitamin A)	Dark green, yellow or orange vegetables and fruit (e.g. carrots, pumpkin, spinach, sweet potatoes, squash or apricots)
Bread and cereal group	4 or more	1 slice of bread 1 oz cereal 4-6 oz cooked cereal, spaghetti or other pasta, or rice.

NUTRITIONAL SUPPORT
All patients should be encouraged to eat a varied and well-balanced diet that includes foods from all the foodgroups (Table 14.6) in amounts sufficient to maintain, or increase, body weight.

To minimise weight loss, and facilitate repair and regeneration of damaged tissues, a high energy, high protein diet is recommended. Items consumed should be selected from as wide a variety of foods as possible since this will help to ensure that vitamin and mineral requirements are met; supplements may be required. Methods of increasing the energy and protein content of the diet are shown in Table 14.7.

Table 14.7   **Some ways of increasing the energy and protein content of the diet**

Energy

Use single or double cream instead of milk

Butter toast when it is hot and will absorb greater amounts of butter

Add cream, evaporated milk or ice cream to milky drinks and deserts

Eat cream soups rather than clear soups

Add mayonnaise, salad dressings, gravies and sauces to meals and sandwiches

Eat potatoes, pasta, rice or bread at least twice a day

Have honey, jam, jelly or syrup with bread or toast and add to milk puddings

Add fruit or full-fat yoghurt to breakfast cereals

Eat between-meal snacks, such as nuts, crisps, sweets, chocolate or dried fruits

Add sugar to deserts and beverages

Fry foods rather than grilling them, eat baked potatoes with butter and/or cheese

Protein

Fortify whole milk with skimmed milk powder, egg or ice cream

Add yoghurt to the daily diet

Eat additional eggs, milk, fish, poultry or eggs

Add eggs and/or cheese to salads, casseroles and sauces or to deserts

---

Modification of the nutrient intake

Many patients cannot meet their nutritional needs through oral intake alone and additional support is needed. A voluntary food intake falling below 80% of the required amounts of energy and protein (Table 14.8) indicates the need for support.

Table 14.8   Energy and protein needs of patients undergoing radiotherapy

Energy		
Females		
	At ideal body weight (IBW)	= IBW x 39.4kcal/kg per day
	With weight loss	= IBW x 44.4kcal/kg per day
Males		
	At ideal body weight (IBW)	= IBW x 44.4kcal/kg per day
	With weight loss	= IBW x 48.4kcal/kg per day

When weight loss exceeds 1kg/week an additional 4.4kcal/kg is added to the daily intake until ideal body weight is reached.

Protein
        IBW x 2g protein/kg/day

The strategy selected for modifying the food intake to ensure an adequate supply of nutrients will depend on the specific feeding problem and the degree of nutritional depletion. The oral route is the preferred method of feeding although this may be difficult when the patient is suffering from anorexia, nausea, taste aberration and dysphagia. Nonetheless, eating must be encouraged by modifying both the food and its presentation; suitable approaches have been discussed in the relevant chapters.

However, individual patients may require particular dietary modifications which can pose difficulties in the hospital environment since the attitude to patient feeding is often surprisingly inflexible and many patients find hospital food unfamiliar and unacceptable. It may be valuable to enlist the help of relatives and/or friends to provide foods which the patient 'fancies' and will enjoy.

There is little doubt that control of those symptoms limiting food intake can help considerably so that regular administration of anti-emetics, analgesics or anti-diarrhoeal medications are simple measures that can be extremely effective.

However, food intake can also be limited by early satiety when the patient feels hungry at the start of a meal but finds he is unable to eat more than a few mouthfuls. In this case, as when caring for those with anorexia, frequent small meals may be more acceptable and nutritional supplements may prove valuable in ensuring an adequate nutrient intake.

The timing of meals deserves some consideration. Many patients complain of a decreased ability to eat as the day progresses, the morning being the best time for eating. The reasons for this are not entirely clear but it may result from a sluggish digestion and reduced rate of gastric emptying due to a reduction in the secretion of gastric enzymes combined with atrophy of both the GI mucosa and the gastric muscle itself (DeWys, 1979). This means that affected patients should be encouraged to eat their largest meal early in the day and to consume frequent, small but nutrient dense snacks or drinks throughout the remainder of the day.

Enteral feeding and nutritional supplements

When patients are unable to eat sufficient food to meet their nutritional needs additional support is essential. This can be achieved in several ways. For example, additional milky drinks, such as milk shakes, can be given to boost the nutrient intake; whole milk provides 160kcal and 8g protein per 200ml. However, despite its value as a nutritional supplement, milk cannot be given to those patients with intestinal damage who are also lactose intolerant or to those who cannot tolerate, digest or absorb a normal diet. In such cases a liquid nutrition formula can be used to overcome some of these difficulties and provide either total or supplemental support.

It is the nurses' role to monitor individual food consumption and, together with other members of the caring team, to decide when alternative methods of feeding are needed. Such modifications may necessitate a simple change in the texture of foods (e.g. a soft or pureed diet) or the need for specialist nutritional approaches.

Liquid formulas may be used as tube feeds, 'sip' feeds or between-meal supplements; they may also be incorporated into 'normal' foods to increase their nutrient density.

Liquid diets may be derived from normal foods (homogenised) or commercially-prepared. Although the latter are more convenient, microbiologically safer and of consistent nutrient composition, those based on normal foods may be more psychologically acceptable to both patient and carer.

The many formulae available make it possible to consider individual needs when selecting feeds. For example, if fat digestion is impaired, a feed.containing readily absorbed fats (medium chain triglycerides) may be given while, for the lactose intolerant, lactose-free formulae can be selected. Complete formulae provide all essential nutrients while modular products provide sources of either protein or carbohydrate and can be used to increase the intake of specific nutrients by increasing the nutrient density of a normal diet. These include products such as Maxipro™ and Maxijul™ (Scientific Hospital Supplies); a variety is now available.

Liquid feeds may be based on either whole protein or protein isolates. Whole protein feeds are derived from eggs, milk or meat and are relatively palatable, less expensive and lower in osmolarity than those based on protein isolates. Since they contain intact and complex nutrients they require normal digestion and absorption so that their use is limited to those patients with normal GI function. Hydrolysed formulae contain 'pre-digested' protein, together with simple carbohydrates and fat, so that they require little digestion and absorption. Their protein is derived from soya beans, milk or eggs. Both types of supplement are available in lactose-free formulations and so can be used for the lactose intolerant patient and are useful adjuncts to the care of the cancer patient. One problem which may be encountered is that most, but not all, supplements currently available are sweet and so may be rejected by many patients, particularly those suffering from taste aberration. Taste fatigue is common; liquid diets rapidly become monotonous and are associated with the lack of satisfaction derived from chewing. In this case, as wide a variety as possible should be offered, including some savoury varieties, if necessary adjusting the flavour to suit the patient.

When supplements are used as the sole source of nutrition the major complications are diarrhoea and cramp-like abdominal pain secondary to the high osmotic load. When the caloric density exceeds 1.5kcal/ml the high solute load can cause dehydration and azotaemia. Both these effects can be overcome by decreasing the tonicity of the feed by adding water and, unless fluid restriction is required, the fluid intake should approximate 1ml/kcal/day. Feeds containing dietary fibre may be useful in helping to maintain gastro-intestinal function; they may also promote feelings of satiety thus overcoming the feelings of hunger often associated with liquid diets.

When precisely defined quantities of nutrients are required

defined formula and elemental diets can be used both of which will meet the basal requirement for both macro- and micronutrients.

Defined formula diets may be based on either hydrolysed protein or free amino acids, simple sugars and very little fat; they are somewhat unpalatable so that various flavouring agents are required to disguise their organic flavour. They cannot, therefore be used in patients with a sensitivity to bitter tastes; in fact, they are rarely given by the oral route.

Elemental diets, based on free amino acids, simple sugars and a minimal amount of fat, have some advantages over other liquid diets as they are totally bulk free and many are almost fat free. Minimal digestion is needed before absorption can take place so that most pancreatic, biliary and small intestinal secretions are not necessary for absorption and, in addition, absorption can occur even when the absorptive surface area is markedly reduced or when the small intestinal mucosa has been disrupted by cancer therapy.

Tube feeding: When oral nutrient intake is inadequate but GI function is normal, tube feeding is the method of choice for providing nutritional support. Compared with parenteral feeding this is more effective in preserving intestinal function and promoting efficient nutrient use (Goodwin and Wilmore, 1988); it is also less expensive and less likely to cause complications. Tube feeding may be used to supply nutrients to patients who have a functional GI tract but who are unable, or unwilling, to take adequate food orally. Feeds may be administered through various routes (Table 14.9).

A nasoenteric tube is preferred when there is no obstruction between the nasopharynx and stomach. The tube selected should be the smallest possible which will permit the passage of the selected feeding formula. They are usually made of silicon-rubber or poly-urethane and do not stiffen or crack even after prolonged use. Most are weighted with either tungsten or mercury which eases its passage into the stomach, jejunum or duodenum. Permanent feeding access is indicated for long-term feeding; this is usually achieved through a tube enterostomy, most commonly a gastrostomy.

Percutaneous gastrostomy under endoscopic control (PEG) is increasingly popular as a means of tube placement for patients who require nutritional support but are poor surgical risks (Payne-James and Silk 1988). When compared with other forms of gastrostomy thisis less costly, the complication rate is low and insertion is relatively straightforward (Taylor and Goodinson-MacLaren, 1992).

Table 14.9   Placement of feeding tubes (from Holmes, 1987)

	Advantages	Disadvantages
Nasogastric	Usually well-tolerated as stomach acts as 'reservoir' holding and releasing feeds at a controlled rate and enhancing absorption thus avoiding dumping syndrome.	The risk of aspiration is high. Contraindicated when patient is vomiting, has GI bleeding or total intestinal obstruction
Nasoduodenal	Risk of aspiration reduced as both lower oesophageal and pyloric sphincters act to inhibit gastric reflux. Feeds can be both digested and absorbed provided correct formula is given.	Dumping syndrome is likely since the stomach is bypassed.
Nasojejunal	Aspiration is extremely unlikely (as above).	Dumping syndrome is common, particularly when hypertonic feeds are given or feeds are administered too quickly.
Oesophagostomy	Usually well tolerated as the stomach is used as 'reservoir'; controlled release of food prevents occurrence of dumping syndrome.	Risk of aspiration is high. Thoracic duct injury may occur.

The most common placement methods are the 'pull-through' (Gauderer-Ponsky) and 'push-through' (Sachs-Vine) techniques. The first requires introducing a guide wire through the abdominal wall. This is pulled out through the mouth by an endoscope, attached to the PEG and then used to pull this into place in the abdominal wall. The latter involves threading the PEG over the guide wire and pushing this through the abdominal wall from inside. In either case, the tube is secured to the external abdominal wall; the tip is positioned in the gastric antrum. Longer tubes may be positioned in the duodenum or jejunum.

Once the PEG is well-established, a gastrostomy button may be inserted into the tract formed by the gastrostomy. Unlike the gastrostomy tube which protrudes and may snag in clothes or interfere with sexual activity this lies almost flush with the skin.

Administration of feeds

Selection of feeding solutions depends on the mode of administration as well as the patient's nutritional condition. Many of the liquid supplements can be given as tube feeds as can defined formula or elemental diets that will meet the basal requirement for all nutrients with the possible exception of vitamin K which can, if necessary, be given by intramuscular injection.

Regardless of the route through which feeds are to be administered, they may be given continuously or by intermittent bolus and either pump-controlled or controlled by gravity. Although continuous feeding is preferred, as it decreases the risk of diarrhoea, bolus feeding is often used, and is certainly more convenient when the patient is treated at home provided that feeds are tolerated and cause no unpleasant symptoms. They have several advantages, such as increased patient mobility and ease of maintenance, and also similarity with the physiological aspects of 'normal' eating. However, uncontrolled bolus feeding may cause nausea, diarrhoea, abdominal cramps and vomiting and, therefore, an increased risk of aspiration. Slow, gravity drip feeds, or those delivered by pump over a 30-40 minute period, are generally better tolerated.

Continuous feeding is usually carried out over a 16-20 hour period to maximise tolerance and increase absorption. It may be carried out overnight for patients in the community. Volumetric pumps provide the safest and most accurate method of continuous infusion and ensure the passage of viscous solutions through a fine bore tube. A pump should always be used when feeding through a duodenostomy or jejunostomy to prevent dumping syndrome. The maximum flow rate should be about 125ml/hr; the rate of administration and the concentration of the solution should be increased gradually over several days to decrease side-effects. Most commercial feeds provide 1-2kcal/ml. However, when caloric density exceeds 1.5kcal/ml, the high osmolarity may cause dehydration and azotaemia. This can be overcome by adding water to dilute the feed; unless fluid restriction is required, intake should approximate 1ml/kcal/day.

The major complications of this method of feeding are diarrhoea and crampy abdominal pain secondary to the high osmotic load. However, whenever enteral feeding is employed, there is a potential risk of aspiration of vomit. This can be prevented by elevating the head of the bed, avoiding night feeds, placing the distal end of the tube beyond the pylorus (although this may increase the risk of dumping syndrome) and carefully evaluating gastric retention. When the residual volume exceeds 75-100ml, feeds should be withheld.

Parenteral feeding

Although parenteral feeding is the least preferred method of nutritional support it must be considered whenever the GI tract is non-functional. When this method of feeding is the only source of nutrients it is referred to as total parenteral nutrition (TPN). It may also be given to support an inadequate oral intake (supplemental parenteral nutrition).

Supplemental nutrition is often given by infusing fluids into a peripheral vein. Such fluids must be isotonic/hypotonic so as to prevent phlebitis and irritation of the vein, and consist of solutions of dextrose, amino acids or lipid emulsion together with vitamins, trace elements and electrolytes. The same nutrients are supplied by TPN but at higher concentrations which are hyperosmolar. Peripheral venous nutrition is usually used on a short term basis (5-7 days) and is useful only for repletion of mild to moderate nutritional depletion when nutrient needs, although greater than normal, are not excessive.

TPN depends on placement of a long-term feeding access device into a large diameter vein, usually the subclavian vein, where the rapid and copious blood flow quickly dilutes the concentrated and hypertonic solutions required to satisfy the patient's nutritional needs without exceeding his daily fluid tolerance. This necessitates placement of a central line

Energy (calories) is usually provided by a carbohydrate such as glucose (dextrose) or fat (lipid) which is a concentrated source of energy providing 9kcal/g compared with the 4kcal/g provided by carbohydrate. Fats are infused in 10% or 20% solution to ensure adequate provision of essential fatty acids thus preventing deficiency. Adequate calories must be given to ensure that administered protein (as amino acids) can be used to synthesise body tissues rather than to supply energy. Minerals, trace elements, vitamins and electrolytes are added to the parenteral solution at the time of preparation. Insulin may also be added since endogenous insulin secretion may be inadequate when hypertonic glucose is administered.

TPN is, however, an expensive procedure requiring continuous monitoring. It carries the risk of serious complications that can be

Nutritional care of the patient undergoing radiotherapy

categorised as mechanical, metabolic and infective (Table 14.10). However, Mullen (1981) reviewed the incidence and severity of complications in cancer patients as compared with non-cancer patients concluding that there was no difference between the two groups so that there are no additional hazards in this group of patients. As a result, TPN is often used to maintain nutritional status in those patients who have lost gastrointestinal function but who are free of disease as well as in the severely malnourished individual for whom active treatment is contemplated. When used for appropriate patients, there is little doubt that TPN improves the response to anticancer therapies and also improves the quality of life (Torosian et al, 1983).

Table 14.10   Potential complications of total parenteral nutrition

Mechanical	Pneumothorax	Injury to brachial plexus
	Haemothorax	Injury to subclavian artery
	Hydrothrorax	Central vein thrombophlebitis
	Thoracic duct injury	Arteriovenous fistula
	Cardiac perforation	Air or catheter embolism
	Catheter misplacement	Endocarditis
	Subclavian haematoma	
Metabolic	Dehydration and electrolyte imbalance	Hyperchloraemic acidosis
		Hyperammonaemia
	Hyperosmolar hyperglycaemia (non-ketotic)	Azotaemia
		Trace element deficiency
	Hyper/hypophosphataemia	Rebound hypoglycaemia on
	Hypocalcaemia	cessation of treatment
	Hypomagnesaemia	
Infective	Entry site - contamination during insertion	
	Catheter 'seeding' from blood-borne or other (distant) infection	
	Contamination of feeding solution	

This technique can also be used at home provided that the patient, and/or his relatives, have been trained to cope. There must also be supportive and regular follow-up of these patients. Use of home TPN can permit a return to a normal life and work thus significantly improving the quality of life.

Psychological aspects of nutritional support

Since nutritional support may have a number of psychological and social consequences the occurrence of which increases with the length of the period of support (Gulledge, 1987) patients may require considerable support and encouragement. Artificial feeding may cause feelings of frustration, loss of control and independence and, for some, suggests a return to childhood; the presence of a feeding tube may cause disgust, anger and concern at alterations in body image This may necessitate significant changes in lifestyle markedly altering family and social activities many of which focus around food and drink (Gulledge, 1987). A loss of libido is common.

PATIENT COMPLIANCE

Regardless which method of feeding is used patient compliance and co-operation is essential if nutritional care and support is to be successful. This means that the patient must understand the reasons for such care. It is also essential that both the patient and his family are aware of the problems that may arise and their possible solutions. Teaching should take place at an early stage in their course of radiotherapy and should continue in conjunction with periodic nutritional assessment. Specific goals should be established; these must be achieved and directed towards a tangible means of feedback, such as body weight or improvement in general well-being.

THE TERMINAL PATIENT

Clearly the patient with cancer, who is also undergoing radiotherapy, is at a considerable risk of malnutrition, problems that may persist long after therapy has been completed. An awareness of these effects, together with an understanding of its cause, will help all members of the caring team to plan appropriate preventive measures.

However, it must be recognised that nutritional support, although it is an important part of the total care of all patients whatever their disease, will not cure cancer although it can improve the patient's response to treatment as well as his quality of life. It can be very disturbing for the patient and his relatives to observe the continuing muscle wasting and physical weakness that accompany starvation so that nutritional support can also play an important supportive role. However, it is of questionable benefit for the patient in whom antineoplastic therapy has failed and who has no realistic expectations of a positive outcome. Thus there comes a time when unwanted nutritional support should not be continued since an extension of life may prolong suffering. It may be more appropriate to suggest that the patient should eat what, if any, food is wanted and that he is given emotional and psychological support and comfort. Nutrition no longer matters; the pleasurable aspects of food and eating should be emphasised with little concern about its quantity or its nutrient content.

REFERENCES

Bernstein IL, Bernstein ID, 1981, Learned food aversions and cancer anorexia, Cancer Treatment Reports, **65** (Suppl), 43-44.

Beutler B, Cerami A, 1986, Cachectin and tumour necrosis factor as two sides of the same biological coin, Nature, **110**, 584-88.

Cooper EH, Stone J, 1979, Acute phase reactant proteins in cancer. In: Klein G, Weinhouse S (Editors), Advances in Cancer Research, Academic Press, New York.

Daly JM, Dudrick SJ, Copeland EM, 1979, Evaluation of nutritional indices as prognostic indicators in the cancer patient, Cancer, **43**, 925-931.

DeWys WD, 1979, Anorexia as a general effect of cancer, Cancer, **43**, 2013-2014.

Durnin JVGA, Fidanza F, 1985, Evaluation of nutritional status, Bibliotheca Nutrition and Dietetics, **35**, 20-30.

Fearon KCH, 1992, The mechanisms and treatment of weight loss in cancer, Proceedings of the Nutrition Society, **51**, 251-265.

Garrow J, 1994, Starvation in Hospital, Letter to the Editor, British Medical Journal, **306**, 934.

Gelin J, Lundholm K, 1992, The metabolic response to cancer, Proceedings of the Nutrition Society, **51**, 279-84.

Gibson RS, 1990, Principles of Nutritional Assessment, Oxford University Press, Oxford.

Goodinson SM, 1987a, Anthropometric assessment of nutritional status, Professional Nurse, **2**, 388-393.

Goodinson SM, 1987b, Biochemical assessment of nutritional status, Professional Nurse, **2**, 8-12.

Gulledge AD, 1987, Psychosocial issues of home parenteral and enteral nutrition, Nutrition in Clinical Practice, **2**, 183-194.

Heber D, Byerly CO, Cheblowski RT, 1985, Metabolic abnormalities in the cancer patient, Cancer, **55** (Suppl), 225-229.

Holland, JCB, Rowland J, Plumb M, 1977, Psychological aspects of anorexia in cancer patients, Cancer Research, **37**, 3425-3428.

Holmes S, 1986, Nutritional needs of medical patients, Nursing

Times, **82** (17), 34-36.

Holmes S, 1987, Artificial feeding, Nursing Times, **83**, 49-58.

Holmes S, Dickerson JWT, 1988, Malignant disease: nutritional implications of disease and treatment, Cancer and Metastasis Reviews, **6**, 357-381.

Holmes S, Dickerson JWT, 1991, Food intake and quality of life in cancer patients, Journal of Nutritional Medicine, **2**, 359-368.

Johnston CA, Keaner TJ, Prudo SM, 1980, Weight loss in patients receiving radical radiation therapy for head and neck cancer: a prospective study, Journal of Parenteral and Enteral Nutrition, **6**, 399-402.

Kawakami M, Cerami A, 1981, Studies of endotoxin-induced decrease in lipoprotein lipase activity, Journal of Experimental Medicine, **154**, 631-39.

Kokal WA, 1985, The impact of antitumour therapy on nutrition, Cancer, **55**, 273-278.

Kruk ZL, 1976, Dopamine and 5-hydroxytryptamine inhibit feeding in rats, Nature, New Biology, **246**, 52-7.

Landel AM, Hammond, WG, Meguid MM, 1985, Aspects of amino acid and protein metabolism in cancer bearing states, Cancer, **55** (Suppl), 230-237.

Leathwood PD, Ashley DV, Moennoz DV, 1986, Anorexia and cachexia in cancer, Nestlé Research News 1985/86, Néstec Ltd., Switzerland.

Lehr D, Goldman W, 1973, Continued pharmacologic analysis of consummatory behaviour in the albino rat, European Journal of Pharmacology, **23**, 197-200.

Mattes RD, Arnold C, Boraas M, 1987, Management of learned food aversion in cancer patients receiving cancer chemotherapy, Cancer Treatment Reports, **71**, 1071-1078.

Morrison SD, 1976, Control of food intake in cancer cachexia: a challenge and a tool, Physiology and Behaviour, **17**, 705-709.

Mullen JL, 1981, Complications of total parenteral nutrition in the cancer patient, Cancer Treatment Reports, **65**, (Supplement 5), 107-115.

Novin D, van der Weele DA, 1977, Visceral involvement in feeding, Progress in Physiology and Psychology, **7**, 193-241.

Ollenschlager G, Konkol K, Modder B, 1988, Indicators for and results of nutritional therapy in cancer patients, Recent Results in Cancer Research, **108**, 172-184.

Padilla G, 1986, Psychological aspects of nutrition and cancer, Surgical Clinics of North America, **66**, 1121-34.

Payne-James JJ, Silk DBA, 1988, Enteral nutrition: background indications and management, Clinical Gastroenterology, **2**, 815-847.

Peck A, Boland J, 1977, Emotional reactions to radiation treatment, Cancer, **40**, 180-184.

Plumb M, Holland J, Park S, Dykstia L, Holmes J, 1976, Depression of symptoms in patients with advanced cancer: a controlled assessment (Abstr) Psychosomatic Medicine, **36**, 459.

Schmale AH, 1979, Psychological aspects of anorexia: areas for study, Cancer, **43**, 2087-92.

Selby P, Hobbs S, Viner C et al, 1987, Tumour necrosis factor in man: clinical and biological observations, British Journal of Cancer, **56**, 803-808.

Shils ME, 1977, Nutritional problems induced by cancer, Medical Clinics of North America, **63**, 1009-1025.

Taylor S, Goodinson-MacLaren S, 1992, Nutritional support: a team approach, Wolfe Publishing Ltd., London.

Torosian MH, Mullen JL, Miller EE, 1983, Enhanced tumour response to cycle specific chemotherapy by parenteral amino acid administration, Journal of Parenteral and Enteral Nutrition, **7**, 337-345.

Torti FM, Dieckmann B, Beutler B et al, 1985, A macrophage factor inhibits adipocyte gene expression: an in vitro model of cachexia, Science, **229**, 867-869.

von Meyendfeldt MF, Chance WT, Fischer JE, 1980, Investigation of serotonergic influence on cancer-induced anorexia, Neuroscience Abstracts, **6**, 525-26.

Wangel AG, Deller DJ, 1966, Malabsorption syndrome associated with carcinoma of the bronchus, Gut, **6**, 73-76.

Wesdorp RIC, Krause R, von Meyendfeldt MF, 1983, Cancer cachexia and its nutritional implications, British Journal of Surgery, **70**, 352-355.

Wright RA, Heymsfield, 1985, Nutritional Assessment, Blackwell Scientific Publications, Oxford.

GLOSSARY OF TERMS

Adjuvant therapy:	Additional treatment, by radiotherapy or chemotherapy, given to destroy any residual cancer cells left behind after surgery.
Afterloading techniques:	An important protective method which enables staff exposure to radiation to be reduced during brachytherapy. Suitable catheters or containers are placed in position; the radioactive source is rapidly inserted using either manual or automatic techniques.
ALARA:	As low as reasonably achievable.
Alopecia:	The absence of hair from skin areas where it is normally present; baldness.
Anaemia:	Reduction, to below normal levels, of the numbers of erythrocytes, quantity of haemoglobin or volume of packed cells in the blood.
Anergy:	State in which the immune system is unresponsive.
Anorexia:	Reduction in, or loss of, appetite for food.
Anthropometry:	The science dealing with measurement of size, weight or proportions of the body (ie. physical measurements).
Ascites:	The effusion and accumulation of serous fluid in the abdominal cavity.
Atomic number:	The number of protons in the nucleus of an atom.
Atomic weight:	The weight of an atom of an element compared with the weight of an atom of hydrogen. It approximates to the number of protons plus the number of neutrons in the nucleus of that atom.
Becquerel:	Measure of the specific activity of a radionuclide. Specifically used to describe the number of atoms of a radioisotope which disintegrate in one second. Now replaces the Curie.
Brachytherapy:	Term used to describe the administration of radiation via a radioactive source placed in, or in close proximity to, the tumour. Achieved by permanent or temporary implantation of a radioactive source in, or immediately adjacent, to the tumour. May also include systemic therapy.
Carcinogen:	A substance which may contribute to the production of

cancer.

Carcinogenic: Capable of causing cancer, or contributing to its cause.

Carcinogenesis: The production of cancer.

Cardiac tamponade: Cardiac compression due to the collection of fluid (e.g. blood) in the pericardial space; intrapericardial effusion.

Cell cycle: Term used to describe the phases of cell replication.

Cell survival curve: Graph obtained by plotting the fraction of a cell population which survives against the dose of radiation received. Used to describe the biological effects of irradiation.

Chemotherapy: The treatment of disease with chemical agents (usually drugs); in the case of cancer therapy refers to cytotoxic drugs.

Cystitis: Condition causing inflammation of the urinary bladder. Characterised by dysuria, frequency of micturition and urgency, often accompanied by low back pain, stress incontinence and, at times, haematuria.

Dental caries: Destructive process which results in decalcification of the tooth enamel and leads to continued destruction of both enamel and dentine and cavitation of the tooth.

Desquamation: Shedding of the epithelial elements, chiefly of the skin in scales or sheets.

DNA: Deoxyribonucleic acid; genetic material (chromosomes) present in the nucleus of all cells and essential if cell replication is to take place.

Dose equivalent: Calculation of the biologically effective dose of radiation which makes allowance for the relative biological effectiveness (RBE) of the radiation involved. (See RBE).

Dumping syndrome: Nausea, weakness, sweating, palpitations, syncope often accompanied by a sensation of warmth and, sometimes, diarrhoea which occurs after food ingestion in patients who have undergone partial gastrectomy.

Dysgeusia: Impaired sense of taste.

Dyspnoea: Laboured or difficult breathing.

Dysuria: Painful or difficult urination.

Electromagnetic radiation:	Type of radiation which is in the form of short length, high energy waves (e.g. X-rays, gamma rays).
Electrons:	Small, light, negatively charged particles which surround the nucleus of an atom.
Epilation:	The removal (loss) of hair from the roots.
Erythropoeisis:	The production of erythrocytes.
Excoriation:	Any superficial loss of substance such as that of the skin produced by scratching.
External therapy:	See teletherapy.
Extravasation:	A discharge or escape of blood/fluid from a vessel into the surrounding tissue.
Fibrosis:	The formation of fibrous tissue.
Film Badge:	Personal dosimeter which enables monitoring of individual exposure to radiation. Reliant on photographic film to provide a record of type and length of exposure.
Free radicals:	Highly reactive molecules having an unpaired electron. In this context, they often arise when water (contained by all biological materials) is subjected to the radiation used in the treatment of cancer.
Geiger Muller counter:	A monitoring device used to measure the amount of radiation present in the environment.
Gray:	The SI unit of absorbed dose of radiation. Defined as 1 joule/kg. Replaces the rad; 1 Gy = 100 rads or 1 Rad = 1 centigray.
Growth fraction:	The fraction of cells in any tissue which are in the state of active division.
Haematemesis:	Vomiting of blood.
Haematocrit:	The volume percentage of erythrocytes in whole blood. Also used to describe the procedure or equipment used in its determination.
Haemopoietic tissue:	Tissue, such as the bone marrow, in which the formation and development of blood cells takes place.
Haemostasis:	The arrest of bleeding either by the physiological processes of vasoconstriction and coagulation or by surgical means. May also be used to describe the interruption of blood flow through any vessel or to any anatomical area.
Half life ($t_{1/2}$):	The time in which the rate of disintegration of a radioactive material drops to half.

Glossary of terms

Hyperaemia: An excess of blood in a part of the body.

Hypercapnia: Abnormal retention of CO_2, with $pH<7.35$ which produces respiratory acidosis.

Hyperfractionation: Radiation therapy in which an accelerated fractionation regime is followed. Relies on delivery of the same total dose in a shortened time; radiation is delivered more than once a day.

Hyperventilation: Abnormally increased pulmonary ventilation resulting in a reduced concentration of carbon dioxide in the bloodstream which, if prolonged, leads to respiratory alkalosis. Blood gases will show decreased pCO_2, an increased pO_2 and an elevated pH (>7.45).

Hypoguesia: Decreased taste sensation.

Hypoventilation: Reduction in the amount of air entering the pulmonary alveoli. Blood gases will show an elevation of pCO_2, a decreased pH (<7.35) and a decreased pO_2 unless the patient is receiving supplemental O_2 therapy when the pO_2 may be satisfactory but CO_2 retention will continue.

Hypoxia: The absence of oxygen; a decrease in oxygen tension.

Immunocompetence: The ability to mount an immune response following exposure to an antigen.

Immunodeficiency: A deficiency of the immune response due to hypo-activity or decreased numbers of lymphoid cells.

Intracavity therapy: Insertion of a radioactive source into a body cavity.

Intraoperative radiotherapy: Delivery of a single, large fraction of radiotherapy to a tumour site following surgical exposure. The surgical procedure is then completed and may be followed by further external radiotherapy.

Interstitial therapy: Treatment with radiation when the radioactive source is applied between the parts or in the interspaces of a tissue.

Inverse square law: A law of physics which states that the intensity of radiation is inversely proportional to the square of the distance from the radioactive source. As a result, the intensity of the irradiation is reduced to a quarter when the distance from the source is doubled (see text).

Ion: An atom or molecule which has gained or lost one or more electrons and acquired a positive (a cation) or negative charge (an anion)

Ion pair: Radiation energy may cause release of an ion and a free electron (charged particle) which, together, form highly reactive ion pairs (see text).

Ionisation: The dissociation of a substance into ions (ie. the process through which electrons are removed and an ion is formed).

Ionising radiation: Radiation is said to be ionising when it is able to disrupt the structure of the material through which it passes causing damage to, or disruption of, the atoms and molecules contained by that material.

Isocentre: The term used to describe the point about which diagnostic or therapeutic equipment rotates.

Isodose curves: These are used to describe the percentage of radiation remaining in a radiation beam at any given depth in normal tissues. Allows anatomical contours to be outlined so that they receive the same dose of irradiation. Used in designing the optimum treatment plan for a specified tumour.

Isotopes: Atoms with the same atomic number but different atomic weights due to the presence of varying numbers of neutrons in the nucleus although the number of protons is the same.

Leucopoenia: A reduction in the number of leucocytes in the blood.

Mucositis: Generalised inflammation of the mucous membranes.

Myelosuppression: Inhibition of bone marrow activity resulting in a decreased production of blood cells and platelets.

Necrosis: Morphological changes indicative of cell death, due to progressive enzymatic degradation. May affect groups of cells or part of an organ.

Nephritis: Inflammation of the kidney which may affect the glomerulus, tubules or interstitial tissues resulting in a focal or diffuse and proliferative disease.

Neutron: An uncharged (neutral) particle present in the nucleus of an atom.

Nuclear disintegration: See radioactive decay.

Nutritional assessment: Means of assessing nutritional status by collecting and interpreting nutrition-related data.

Nutritional status: Extent to which an individual's physiological need for nutrients is met by the food he is (or has been) eating.

221

Glossary of terms

Oocytes:	Immature ovum (female reproductive or germ cells).
Oophoropexy:	Surgical procedure involving elevation of the ovaries and fixing to the abdominal wall.
Osteoradionecrosis:	Necrosis of the bone due to excessive exposure to ionising radiation.
Palliate:	Relieve symptoms.
Palliative care:	Care directed towards the relief of distressing symptoms.
Pancreatitis:	Inflammation of the pancreas. Characterised by abdominal pain and vomiting, incomplete digestion and absorption. Steatorrheoa and diarrhoea will occur if the condition is chronic. Hypovolaemia and shock may be present in an acute episode.
Parasthesiae:	Unpleasant sensations of numbness or heaviness; usually affects a limb or limbs.
Petechiae:	Tiny haemorrhagic spots due to intradermal or submucosal bleeding.
Photons:	A particle (quantum) of radiant energy
Pneumonitis:	Inflammation of pulmonary tissue accompanied by a dry, persistent cough, dyspnoea on exertion, weakness and fatigue and, occasionally, pyrexia.
Purpura:	Purplish/brownish red discolouration of the skin easily visible through the epidermis due to haemorrhage into the tissues.
Radiation-absorbed dose:	Measure of the energy deposited by any form of ionising radiation. Unit of measurement = Gray (see Gray).
Radiation syndrome:	Generalised effects resulting from exposure to radiation. Includes fatigue, lethargy, nausea and vomiting.
Radioactivity:	Spontaneous emission of radiation following nuclear disintegration during radioactive decay. Results in emission of α, β or γ radiation from atomic nucleii (see below).
Radioactive decay:	Process of disintegration of the nucleus of a radioactive atom during which radiation is released.
Radiocurable:	Curable by irradiation.
Radioepithelite:	White/yellow pseudomembrane developing in the mouth following radiation-induced mucositis.
Radioisotope:	A radioactive isotope (see isotope).

Radiolabelled antibodies: Antibodies, usually monoclonal antibodies, to which a radioactive substance has been attached. These bind to tumour-associated antigens leading to the possibility of targeted therapy in which radiation is delivered directly to the target tumour.

Radioprotectors: Compounds that can protect well-oxygenated (non-tumour) cells while having a limited effect on hypoxic tumour cells.

Radioresistance: Resistance of cells/tissues to radiation.

Radioresponsive: Reacting favourably to irradiation.

Radiosensitisers: Substances (e.g. drugs) which are used to increase sensitivity to radiation in hypoxic cells. Appear to act by promoting fixation of free radicals produced by radiation-induced damage rendering affected molecule incapable of repair..

Radiosensitivity: Sensitivity to radiant energy (radiation).

Relative biological effectiveness: Because different types of radiation lose energy at different rates RBE allows comparison of a dose of test radiation with a dose of standard radiation producing the same biological effect. Expressed by the formula:

$$RBE = \frac{\text{Dose of standard radiation which produces given biological effects}}{\text{Dose of test radiation which produces same biological effect}}$$

RNA: Ribonucleic acid found in the nucleus of all cells. Essential for protein synthesis.

Scintillation counter: Instrument capable of detecting low energy radiation. Primarily used in the laboratory setting.

Sealed sources: Solid radioisotopes used to deliver radiation in close proximity to the tumour (brachytherapy).

Sievert: Term used to describe the dose equivalent.

Specific activity: The number of particles emitted per second by a given weight of a radioactive element.

Spermatogonia: An undifferentiated male germ cell which originates in a seminal tubule and divides to form two spermatocytes.

Systemic therapy: Administration of radioactive material in liquid form (as a suspension or a colloid) using a variety of methods of administration (e.g. ingestion, infusion into vascular/lymphatic system or injection into a body cavity).

Target area (target volume):	Area to be treated with irradiation which includes the tumour and an adequate safety margin as delineated by the treatment plan.
Teletherapy:	Treatment in which the source of the therapeutic agent (e.g. radiation) is sited at a distance from the body (ie. external beam therapy).
Teratogenic effects:	Production of alterations/changes in a developing embryo or foetus.
Therapeutic ratio:	Relationship between the dose of radiation which can be tolerated by the normal tissues adjacent to the tumour and that required to destroy malignant cells.
Thermoluminescent dosimeter:	Personal dosimeter which enables determination of the amount of radiation exposure. Sensitive but expensive and, unlike film badge does not provide a permanent record or detailed information about the quality of the radiation to which the user has been exposed.
Threshold resistance:	Term used to describe the initial resistance to the effects of radiation.
Thrombocytopoenia:	A quantitative decrease in the number of circulating platelets.
Tumour lethal dose:	Dose of radiation which carries a 95% probability of control or cure of malignant disease.
Unit of absorbed dose:	See Gray.
Unsealed sources:	Soluble radioisotopes used to treat malignant disease. May be administered into a cavity (e.g. pleural cavity) or intravenously.
Xerostomia:	Dryness of the oral cavity due to lack of normal secretions (saliva).

INDEX

225

Index

Index